Procedure Checklists to Accompany
Craven & Hirnle's

Fundamentals of Nursing

FOURTH EDITION

Procedure Checklists to Accompany

Craven & Hirnle's

Fundamentals of Nursing

HUMAN HEALTH AND FUNCTION

FOURTH EDITION

Elisa Swisher Sauer, MSN, RN
Former Assistant Dean for Health Services
Director, Nursing Programs
Reading Area Community College
Reading, Pennsylvania

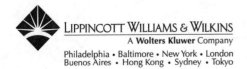

LIPPINCOTT WILLIAMS & WILKINS
A **Wolters Kluwer** Company
Philadelphia • Baltimore • New York • London
Buenos Aires • Hong Kong • Sydney • Tokyo

Acquisitions Editor: Elizabeth Nieginski
Managing Editor: Doris Wray

Senior Project Editor: Rosanne Hallowell
Senior Production Manager: Helen Ewan
Managing Editor / Production: Erika Kors
Art Director: Carolyn O'Brien
Manufacturing Manager: William Alberti
Compositor: Lippincott Williams & Wilkins
Printer: Victor Graphics

9 8 7 6 5 4 3

ISBN 0-7817-3882-2

Care has been taken to confirm the accuracy of the information presented and to describe generally accepted practices. However, the authors, editors, and publisher are not responsible for errors or omissions or for any consequences from application of the information in this book and make no warranty, express or implied, with respect to the content of the publication.

The authors, editors, and publisher have exerted every effort to ensure that drug selection and dosage set forth in this text are in accordance with the current recommendations and practice at the time of publication. However, in view of ongoing research, changes in government regulations, and the constant flow of information relating to drug therapy and drug reactions, the reader is urged to check the package insert for each drug for any change in indications and dosage and for added warnings and precautions This is particularly important when the recommended agent is a new or infrequently employed drug.

Some drugs and medical devices presented in this publication have Food and Drug Administration (FDA) clearance for limited use in restricted research settings. It is the responsibility of the health care provider to ascertain the FDA status of each drug or device planned for use in his or her clinical practice.

Preface

This checklist manual has been developed to provide faculty and students with a portable handbook to the procedures in the text *Fundamentals of Nursing: Human Health and Function.* These checklists may be removed and used during supervision of students' performance of procedures. They may be modified to meet the needs of the situation, if desired. Students will find these checklists helpful when reviewing for the performance of various procedures.

The procedures in the checklists follow the steps of the procedures in the book with some minor modifications. Where there are subsets of procedures—for example, measuring weight—a separate checklist is provided for each procedure. In these instances, some of the introductory steps remain the same in each procedure but the subsequent steps vary. When this occurs, the procedure step number will deviate from the checklist step number even though the content is the same. In other instances the steps "Gather equipment," "Wash hands," "Document procedure and observations" has been added for continuity when these did not appear in the procedure in the text.

It is hoped that this manual will be useful to you, the faculty, as you teach and supervise students in the nursing classroom laboratory or in a clinical experience. It is also hoped that you, the students, will find the checklists useful in preparation for clinical experience.

Procedure Checklists

Name _Fallen_   Date _8/31/05_

Unit _____   Position _____

Instructor/Evaluator: _____   Position _____

Excellent	Satisfactory	Needs Practice	PROCEDURE 24-1 **MEASURING WEIGHT**	Comments
			Goal: Provide baseline data from which to assess total fluid balance or nutritional status, and determine drug dosages.	
	✓		1. Have client void before weighing.	_(handwritten)_
	✓		2. Have client wear same clothing for each weight measurement, and remove slippers or shoes.	_8/31/05_
	✓		3. Place protective paper or cloth on scale.	
	✓		4. Check that scale registers zero. Adjust as necessary.	
			Standing Scale	
	✓		1. Assist client onto center of scale platform. Instruct client not to lean or hold onto supports.	
	✓		2. Read digital display or adjust counterweights to determine client's weight.	
	✓		3. Assist client from scale, and record weight in client's record.	
			Chair Scale	
			1. Place scale beside client and lock wheels.	
			2. Transfer client onto chair. If arm of chair is removable, unlock and remove before transfer. Lock back into place after transfer.	
			3. Read digital display or adjust counterweights to determine client's weight.	
			4. Transfer client back to bed or wheelchair.	
			5. Clean scale according to agency policy. Return to proper location and plug in. Keep battery charged for next use.	
			Bed Scale	
			1. Elevate client's bed to level of stretcher scale.	
			2. With one or two assistants, turn client on side with back toward the scale.	
			3. Roll scale toward bed, lock wheels in place, and lower stretcher onto bed.	
			4. Position folded stretcher under client. Roll client onto stretcher.	

PROCEDURE 24-1
MEASURING WEIGHT (Continued)

Excellent	Satisfactory	Needs Practice		Comments

5. Attach stretcher arms to stretcher, and gradually elevate stretcher about 2 inches above mattress surface. Inform client before elevating. Reassure that he or she will not fall, but head may feel lower than body.

6. Determine that stretcher is not touching any equipment. Lift drains and tubing away from stretcher.

7. Read digital display for client's weight.

8. Gradually lower stretcher to bed. Remove stretcher arms and transfer client off stretcher. Remove stretcher.

9. Unlock bed scale wheels and move away from bed.

10. Assist client to comfortable position.

11. Clean stretcher and scale according to agency policy.

12. Record weight and note any extra linen or equipment weighed with the client.

Name _____ Date _____

Unit _____ Position _____

Instructor/Evaluator: _____ Position _____

Excellent	Satisfactory	Needs Practice	PROCEDURE 24-2 **ASSESSING THE NEUROLOGIC SYSTEM**	
			Goal: To obtain baseline information about the client's neurologic status.	**Comments**
___	___	___	1. Wash hands.	
___	___	___	2. Assemble equipment.	
			Cognitive-Sensory Assessment	
___	___	___	1. Assess the client's level of consciousness by asking direct questions that require a verbal response. Note appropriateness of response and emotional status.	
___	___	___	2. Evaluate client's speech patterns.	
___	___	___	3. Observe general appearance: hygiene, appropriateness of clothing to setting and weather.	
___	___	___	4. If responses are inappropriate, ask direct questions related to person, place, and time (e.g., "What is your name?" "Where are you right now?" "What city do you live in?" "What day is this?"). Be sure a communication or language problem is not causing client's inappropriate response.	
___	___	___	5. If client does not respond or inappropriately responds to orientation questions, give simple commands (e.g., "Squeeze my fingers" or "Wiggle your toes"). If there is no response to verbal commands, test response to painful stimuli by applying firm pressure on client's sternum or finger nailbed with your thumb. Avoid pinching client's skin to elicit a pain response.	
___	___	___	6. Document level of consciousness objectively by stating specific client responses to verbal or tactile stimulation. (Use of Glasgow Coma Scale helps charting of frequent level of consciousness testing.)	
___	___	___	7. Assess function of cranial nerves.	
___	___	___	a. I (Olfactory)—Ask client to identify different mild aromas, like vanilla, coffee, chocolate, cloves.	
___	___	___	b. II (Optic)—Ask client to read Snellen chart.	
___	___	___	c. III (Oculomotor) —Assess pupil reaction to penlight (pupillary reflex).	

Excellent	Satisfactory	Needs Practice		Comments
——	——	——	d. III—Assess direction of gaze by holding finger 18 inches from client's face. Ask client to follow finger up and down and side to side (extraocular eye movements).	
——	——	——	e. IV (Trochlear)—Assess direction of gaze when testing cranial nerve II.	
——	——	——	f. V (Trigeminal)—Lightly touch cotton swab to lateral sclera of eye to elicit blink.	
——	——	——	g. V (cont.)—Measure sensation of touch and pain on face with cotton wisp and pin.	
——	——	——	h. VI (Abducens)—Assess direction of gaze when testing cranial nerve III.	
——	——	——	i. VII (Facial)—Ask client to smile, frown, raise eyebrows.	
——	——	——	j. VII (cont.)—Ask client to identify different tastes on tip and sides of tongue: sugar, salt, lemon juice.	
——	——	——	k. VIII (Auditory)—Assess ability to hear spoken word.	
——	——	——	l. IX (Glossopharyngeal)—Ask client to identify different tastes on back of tongue (as in j).	
——	——	——	m. IX (cont.)—Place a tongue blade on posterior tongue while client says "ah" to elicit gag response.	
——	——	——	n. IX (cont.)—Ask client to move tongue up and down and side to side.	
——	——	——	o. X (Vagus)—Assess with cranial nerve IX by observing palate and pharynx move as client says "ah."	
——	——	——	p. XI (Spinal accessory)—Ask client to turn head side to side and shrug shoulders against resistance from examiner's hands.	
——	——	——	q. XII (Hypoglossal)—Ask client to stick out tongue to midline, then move it side to side.	
——	——	——	8. Assess sensory pathways. a. Client's eyes should be closed during all sensory tests.	
——	——	——	b. Apply stimuli to skin in a random unpredictable order while comparing one side of body to the other.	
——	——	——	c. Client should verbally state when he or she feels a particular stimulus. If an area of altered sensation is detected, note which spinal cord segment is affected by referring to a dermatome chart.	
——	——	——	9. Test pain sensation first by lightly touching pointed end and then blunt end of sterile toothpick to proximal and distal aspects of arms and legs.	

ASSESSING THE NEUROLOGIC SYSTEM (Continued)

Excellent	Satisfactory	Needs Practice		Comments

10. Test temperature sensation by touching skin with vials of hot and then cold water. Client should identify hot versus cold sensation.

11. Lightly stroke proximal and distal aspects of client's arms and legs with a cotton ball or cotton applicator. Ask client to state when and where each stroke is felt.

12. Apply a vibrating tuning fork to the distal interphalangeal joint of fingers and great toe. Ask client to state what is felt and when it stops. If client does not feel vibration, move tuning fork to next joint until sensation is felt.

Activity and Mobility Assessment

1. Inspect arm and leg muscles for atrophy, tremors, fasciculations, or other abnormal movements.

2. Assess strength of specific muscle groups by having client extend or flex individual joints against resistance provided by examiner's hands. Test biceps, triceps, wrist and leg muscles, and ankle. Evaluate for symmetry of same muscle groups.

3. Ask client to close eyes and hold arms in front of body with palms up. Hold position for 30 seconds and observe for pronation of hands or drifting of arms. Notice weaknesses on one or both sides.

4. Evaluate coordination and balance:

    a. Perform a series of rapid alternating movements (RAMs).

    (1) Have client pat upper thigh by rapidly alternating palm and back of hand.

    (2) With dominant hand, have client touch thumb to each finger on that hand as quickly as possible.

    (3) Have client use dominant forefinger to first touch your forefinger, then his or her nose. Instruct client to repeat this as many times as fast as he or she can.

    b. Romberg test—Ask client to stand with feet together, arms at sides. Have client maintain this position for 30 seconds with eyes open, then 30 seconds with eyes closed. Assess for swaying. Stay close to client in case he or she begins to fall.

    c. Ask client to walk across room. Observe gait for symmetry, rhythm, limping, shuffling, or other abnormalities.

PROCEDURE 24-2
ASSESSING THE NEUROLOGIC SYSTEM (Continued)

Excellent	Satisfactory	Needs Practice		Comments
——	——	——	5. Assess deep tendon reflexes (biceps, triceps, patellar, Achilles) using the following technique:	
——	——	——	a. Compare symmetry of reflex on each side of body.	
——	——	——	b. Extremity to be tested should be completely relaxed and slightly extended.	
——	——	——	c. Reflex hammer is held loosely and allowed to swing freely into an arc.	
——	——	——	d. Tap tendon briskly.	
——	——	——	e. Document reflexes by grading responses 0 to 4+ on a stick figure, comparing bilaterally:	
——	——	——	0: no response	
——	——	——	1+: diminished reflex	
——	——	——	2+: normal	
——	——	——	3+: brisker than normal	
——	——	——	4+: hyperactive	
——	——	——	f. In newborn and infant, assess rooting, sucking, Moro, and tonic neck reflexes.	
——	——	——	6. Document all findings according to agency policy.	

Name _____ Date _____

Unit _____ Position _____

Instructor/Evaluator: _____ Position _____

Excellent	Satisfactory	Needs Practice	PROCEDURE 24-3 **AUSCULTATING HEART SOUNDS**	
			Goal: To assess normal and abnormal functioning of the heart valves and to detect cardiac problems.	**Comments**
___	___	___	1. Wash hands.	
___	___	___	2. Assist client to supine position, lifting gown to expose chest. May reexamine client in upright sitting position and in a left lateral position.	
___	___	___	3. Warm diaphragm of stethoscope by holding between hands for a few moments.	
___	___	___	4. Listen in mitral area using the diaphragm. Identify first and second heart sounds. Count heart rate, noting whether rhythm is regular or irregular. If irregular, count heart rate for 1 full minute.	
___	___	___	5. Listen in aortic area using the diaphragm. Concentrate first on S_1, then S_2, noting if splitting occurs. Shift concentration to systole and then diastole. Listen for extra sounds, such as murmurs.	
___	___	___	6. Listen in pulmonic area still using only the diaphragm. Concentrate on S_1, S_2, systole, and then diastole. Compare loudness of S_2 in the aortic and pulmonic areas.	
___	___	___	7. Move the diaphragm and listen to the tricuspid and mitral areas.	
___	___	___	8. Return to aortic area. Listen in aortic area, using bell of stethoscope. Concentrate on S_1, S_2, systole, and diastole.	
___	___	___	9. Repeat same process, using the bell in pulmonic, tricuspid, and mitral areas. Especially in mitral area, concentrate during diastole to detect presence of a third or fourth heart sound. To increase ability to hear S_3 or mitral murmur, have client lie on left side while auscultating with bell. An S_3 often disappears when client sits up.	
___	___	___	10. Replace client's clothes. Assist to comfortable position.	
___	___	___	11. Record findings, describing intensity, quality, and location of sounds.	

Name _____   Date _____

Unit _____   Position _____

Instructor/Evaluator: _____   Position _____

Excellent	Satisfactory	Needs Practice	PROCEDURE 24-4 **AUSCULTATING BREATH SOUNDS**	Comments
			Goal: To assess breath sounds accurately.	
___	___	___	1. Wash hands.	
___	___	___	2. Assist client to upright sitting position, removing gown to expose chest.	
___	___	___	3. Warm diaphragm of stethoscope by holding between hands for a short time.	
___	___	___	4. Ask client to breathe deeply and slowly through mouth.	
			Auscultate Anterior Chest	
___	___	___	1. Place diaphragm of stethoscope about 1 inch below the middle of the right clavicle, making sure it lies between the ribs. Listen to one full inspiration and exhalation. Repeat the process at the corresponding site on the left side.	
___	___	___	2. Note normal and adventitious breath sounds at each point on the chest as you proceed.	
___	___	___	3. Move stethoscope downward about 1.5 to 2 inches along midclavicular line. Note sounds; move stethoscope laterally to opposite side.	
___	___	___	4. Move stethoscope downward another inch or two along midclavicular line to fifth intercostal space; note sounds and then move to same spot on opposite side of chest.	
			Auscultate Posterior Chest	
___	___	___	1. Instruct client to lean forward and cross arms in front.	
___	___	___	2. Auscultate area 2 inches below shoulders and 2 inches to right of spine. Note sounds, and move to corresponding point on left.	
___	___	___	3. Move stethoscope directly downward 2 or 2.5 inches. Note sounds, then move stethoscope laterally and listen on right.	
___	___	___	4. Repeat process, moving downward 2 to 2.5 inches. Listen to corresponding opposite side.	
___	___	___	5. Move stethoscope downward to area just below scapula. Listen on right and left. Listen laterally along lower rib cage.	
___	___	___	6. Replace client's clothes and assist to comfortable position.	
___	___	___	7. Discuss findings with client.	
___	___	___	8. Record assessment findings, being specific as to the description and location of adventitious sounds.	

Name _____ Date _____

Unit _____ Position _____

Instructor/Evaluator: _____ Position _____

Excellent	Satisfactory	Needs Practice	PROCEDURE 24-5 **AUSCULTATING BOWEL SOUNDS**	
			Goal: To determine presence or absence of intestinal peristalsis.	**Comments**
___	___	___	1. Wash hands and warm stethoscope diaphragm.	
___	___	___	2. Ask client when he or she last ate.	
___	___	___	3. Have client urinate before the examination.	
___	___	___	4. Assist client to a supine position with abdomen exposed.	
___	___	___	5. Visually divide the abdomen into four quadrants using the umbilicus as the central crossing landmark.	
___	___	___	6. Place stethoscope diaphragm in each of the four quadrants of the abdomen. Listen for pitch, frequency, and duration of bowel sounds at each site.	
___	___	___	7. If bowel sounds are not heard, listen for 3 to 5 minutes in all quadrants before concluding that they are absent.	
___	___	___	8. Proceed with rest of physical examination, or cover client's abdomen and assist to comfortable position.	
___	___	___	9. Document findings.	

Name _Fallan Pryor_   Date _8/31/05_

Unit _____   Position _____

Instructor/Evaluator: _____   Position _____

Excellent	Satisfactory	Needs Practice	PROCEDURE 25-1 **ASSESSING BODY TEMPERATURE**	Comments
			Goal: To obtain baseline data for comparing future measurements or to assess for temperature alterations.	
			Assessing Oral Temperature With an Electronic Thermometer	
—	—	—	1. Wash hands. Identify client and explain the procedure.	
—	—	—	2. Remove electronic thermometer from battery pack, and remove temperature probe from unit, noting digital display of temperature on screen (usually 34°C or 94°F).	
—	—	—	3. Securely attach disposable cover over temperature probe.	
—	—	—	4. Hold probe in sublingual pocket of client's mouth.	
—	—	—	5. Wait for a beep (usually 10-20 seconds), which indicates the estimated temperature. Watch to see if temperature continues to rise. When it stops, remove probe from client's mouth, noting the temperature displayed on the unit.	
—	—	—	6. Displace probe cover by pressing the probe release button as you hold the probe over a waste container.	
—	—	—	7. Return probe to storage place within the unit and the thermometer to the battery pack.	
—	—	—	8. Record temperature on vital sign documentation record. Discuss findings with client if appropriate.	
			Assessing Rectal Temperature With an Electronic Thermometer	
—	—	—	1. Wash hands. Don clean gloves. Identify client and explain procedure.	
—	—	—	2. Remove rectal (red) electronic thermometer from battery pack, and remove temperature probe from unit, noting digital display of temperature on screen.	
—	—	—	3. Securely attach the disposable cover over the temperature probe.	
—	—	—	4. Close bedroom door or bed curtains. Assist client to Sims' position with upper leg flexed. Expose only anal area.	
—	—	—	5. Apply water-soluble lubricant liberally to thermometer probe tip.	
—	—	—	6. Separate client's buttocks with one gloved hand.	

Excellent	Satisfactory	Needs Practice		

ASSESSING BODY TEMPERATURE (Continued)

Comments

7. Ask client to take a deep, slow breath. Insert thermometer into anus in direction of umbilicus 0.5 inch for an infant and 1.5 inches for an adult. Do not force.

8. Hold in place until beep is heard. Obtain reading.

9. Displace probe cover by pressing the probe release button as you hold the probe over a waste container. Remove gloves and wash hands.

10. Return probe to storage place within the unit and the thermometer to the battery pack.

11. Record temperature on vital signs documentation record. Discuss findings with client if appropriate.

Assessing Temperature Using a Tympanic Membrane Thermometer

1. Wash hands. Identify client and explain procedure.

2. Remove tympanic thermometer from recharging base, and attach tympanic probe cover to sensor unit.

3. Insert probe into ear canal, making sure the probe fits snugly. Avoid forcing probe too deeply into ear. Pulling on pinna may help straighten ear canal, which permits better exposure of tympanic membrane. Rotate probe handle toward the jawline.

4. Activate the thermometer, and watch for the temperature readout, which is usually displayed within 2 seconds. Remove thermometer.

5. Eject sensor probe cover directly into waste container, and return tympanic thermometer to base for recharging. Store away from temperature extremes.

6. Record temperature on vital signs documentation record. Discuss findings with client if appropriate.

riley rn
8/31/05

Name *Fallan Pryor*

Date _____

Unit _____

Position _____

Instructor/Evaluator: _____

Position _____

Excellent	Satisfactory	Needs Practice	

PROCEDURE 25-2
OBTAINING A PULSE

Goal: To obtain baseline measurement of heart rate and rhythm.

Comments

Obtaining a Radial Pulse

1. Wash hands. Identify client and explain procedure.
2. Position client comfortably with forearm across chest or at side with wrist extended.
3. Place fingertips of your first three fingers along the groove at base of thumb on client's wrist.
4. Press against radial artery to obliterate pulse, then gradually release pressure until pulsations are felt.
5. Assess pulse for regularity and strength.
6. If pulse is not easily palpable, use Doppler:
   a. Apply conducting gel to end of probe or to radial site.
   b. Press "on" button and place probe against skin on pulse site. Reposition slightly using firm pressure until pulsating sound is heard.
7. If pulse is regular, count pulse for 30 seconds and multiply by two. If pulse is irregular, count for 1 full minute. Count initial pulse as zero.
8. Record pulse on vital signs record.

Obtaining an Apical Pulse

1. Wash hands, identify client, and explain the procedure.
2. Position client in supine or sitting position with sternum and left chest exposed.
3. Warm diaphragm of stethoscope by holding in palm of hand for 5 to 10 seconds.
4. Insert the earpieces of stethoscope into ears, and place diaphragm over apex of client's heart.
5. Assess heartbeat for regularity and dysrhythmias.
6. If rhythm is regular, count the heartbeat for 30 seconds and multiply by two. Count for 1 full minute if rhythm is irregular. Count initial pulse as zero.

Excellent	Satisfactory	Needs Practice	

Comments

passed
N Anderson RNMSN
8/31/05

7. Replace client's gown, and assist client to return to a comfortable position.

8. Share results of assessment with client, if appropriate.

9. Document pulse on vital signs record. Specify in documentation that an apical pulse was obtained.

Name _____ Date _____

Unit _____ Position _____

Instructor/Evaluator: _____ Position _____

Excellent	Satisfactory	Needs Practice	PROCEDURE 25-3 **ASSESSING RESPIRATIONS**	Comments
			Goal: To assess respiratory status by evaluating rate and quality.	
—	—	—	1. Wash hands and identify client.	*passed* N Anderson RN MSN 8/31/05
—	—	—	2. After assessment of pulse, keep fingers resting on client's wrist, and observe or feel the rising and falling of chest with respiration. If client is asleep, gently place hand on client's chest to feel chest movement. **Do not** explain procedure to client.	
—	—	—	3. When one complete cycle of inspiration and expiration has been observed, look at second hand of watch and count the number of complete cycles. If rate is regular in an adult, count 30 seconds and multiply by two. In children under 2 years of age or adults with irregular rate, count for 1 full minute.	
—	—	—	4. If respirations are shallow and difficult to count, observe at the sternal notch.	
—	—	—	5. Note depth and rhythm of respiratory cycle.	
—	—	—	6. Discuss findings with client, if applicable.	
—	—	—	7. Document respiratory rate, depth, rhythm, and character.	

NA

Name __F-allan Pryor_____   Date _____

Unit _____   Position _____

Instructor/Evaluator: _____   Position _____

Excellent	Satisfactory	Needs Practice	PROCEDURE 25-4 **OBTAINING BLOOD PRESSURE**	Comments
			Goal: To evaluate the client's hemodynamic status by obtaining information about cardiac output, blood volume, peripheral vascular resistance, and arterial wall elasticity and to obtain baseline measurement of blood pressure.	
	✓		1. Wash hands, and identify client. Explain procedure to client. Assist client to a comfortable position with forearm supported at heart level and palm up.	
	✓		2. Expose upper arm completely.	
	✓		3. Wrap deflated cuff snugly around upper arm with center of bladder over brachial artery. Lower border of cuff is 2 cm above antecubital space in an adult, nearer the antecubital space in an infant.	
	✓		4. If using mercury manometer, the manometer is vertical and at eye level.	
	✓		5. Palpate brachial or radial artery with fingertips. Close valve on pressure bulb, and inflate cuff until pulse disappears. Inflate 30 mm Hg higher. Slowly release valve, and note reading when pulse reappears.	
	✓		6. Fully deflate cuff, and wait 1 to 2 minutes.	
	✓		7. Place stethoscope ear pieces in ears. Repalpate the brachial artery, and place stethoscope diaphragm or bell over site.	
	✓		8. Close bulb valve by turning clockwise. Inflate cuff to 30 mm Hg above reading where brachial pulse disappeared.	
	✓		9. Slowly release valve so pressure drops about 2 to 3 mm Hg/s.	
	✓		10. Identify manometer reading when first clear Korotkoff sound is heard.	
	✓		11. Continue to deflate, and note reading when sound muffles or dampens (fourth Korotkoff) and when it disappears (fifth Korotkoff).	
	✓		12. Deflate cuff completely and remove from client's arm.	
	✓		13. Record blood pressure. Record systolic and diastolic in the form 130/80. If three readings are to be recorded, use the form 130/80/40. Abbreviate RA or LA to indicate right or left arm measurement.	
	✓		14. Assist client to comfortable position, and discuss findings with client, if appropriate.	

Name _Fallon Pry_____   Date _11/2/05_____

Unit _____   Position _____

Instructor/Evaluator: _____   Position _____

PROCEDURE 25-5
ASSESSING FOR ORTHOSTATIC HYPOTENSION

Excellent	Satisfactory	Needs Practice	**Goal:** To assess the compensatory status of the cardiovascular and autonomic nervous systems to changes in body position.	**Comments**
—	—	—	1. Wash hands. Identify client and explain procedure.	
—	—	—	2. Position client supine with head of bed flat for 10 minutes.	
—	—	—	3. Check and record supine blood pressure and pulse. Keep blood pressure cuff attached.	
—	—	—	4. Assist client to a sitting position with legs dangling over the edge of bed. Wait 2 minutes and check blood pressure and pulse rate.	
—	—	—	5. Assist client to standing position. Wait 2 minutes and check blood pressure and pulse rate. Be alert to signs and symptoms of dizziness.	
—	—	—	6. Assist client back to comfortable position.	
—	—	—	7. Record measurements and any symptoms that accompany the postural change.	
—	—	—	8. Discuss findings with client, if appropriate.	

Name _Fallan Pryor_   Date _____

Unit _____   Position _____

Instructor/Evaluator: _____   Position _____

			PROCEDURE 26-1	

Handwashing

Excellent	Satisfactory	Needs Practice	**Goal:** To prevent transfer of microorganisms from healthcare personnel to client and from client to healthcare personnel.	**Comments**
___	___	___	1. Remove all rings except a plain wedding band. Push watch 4 to 5 inches above wrist.	
___	___	___	2. Turn on the water and adjust temperature to warm. Do not splash water or lean against the wet sink.	
___	___	___	3. Hold hands lower than elbows, and thoroughly wet hands and lower arms under running water.	
___	___	___	4. Apply soap and rub palms, wrists, and back of hands firmly with circular movements. Interlace fingers and thumbs, moving hands back and forth. Continue using plenty of lather and friction for 15 to 30 seconds on each hand. Timing of scrub may vary depending on purpose of wash and the amount of contamination.	
___	___	___	5. Clean under fingernails using fingernails of other hand and additional soap. Use orangewood stick if available.	
___	___	___	6. Rinse hands and wrists thoroughly with hands held lower than forearms.	
___	___	___	7. Dry hands and arms thoroughly with paper towel, wiping from fingertips toward forearm. Discard in proper receptacle.	
___	___	___	8. Turn off water using clean, dry paper towel on faucets.	

Name _____   Date _____

Unit _____   Position _____

Instructor/Evaluator: _____   Position _____

PROCEDURE 26-2

SURGICAL HAND SCRUB

Goal: To remove as many microorganisms from the hands as possible before a sterile procedure to decrease the risk of infection for high-risk groups.

Excellent	Satisfactory	Needs Practice		Comments
___	___	___	1. Remove rings. Apply surgical attire (scrubs, shoe cover, cap or hood, face mask and protective eye wear).	
___	___	___	2. Wash and rinse hands for initial wash.	
___	___	___	3. Open disposable brush impregnated with antimicrobial soap, and adjust water temperature to warm using water control lever.	
___	___	___	4. Wet hands and arms. Keep elbows bent so that hands remain higher than elbows. Water will flow down hands and off elbows.	
___	___	___	5. Use nail stick or cleaner to clean under nails of both hands.	
___	___	___	6. Wet scrub brush or apply antibacterial soap if not already impregnated in the brush.	
___	___	___	7. *Anatomic timed scrub:* Starting with the fingertips, scrub each anatomic area (nails, fingers each side and web space, palmar surface, dorsal surface, and forearm) for the designated amount of time according to agency policy (usually about 5 minutes). Scrub vigorously using vertical strokes. Repeat with other hand.	
			OR	
			Counted brush stroke method: Starting with the fingertips, scrub each anatomic area (nails, fingers each side and web space, palmar surface, dorsal surface, and forearm) for the designated number of strokes according to agency policy. Scrub vigorously using vertical strokes. Repeat with other hand.	
___	___	___	8. Do not touch faucet, clothing, or other objects. Avoid splashing. Rinse hands thoroughly under warm running water, keeping hands elevated to allow water to drain off at the flexed elbow.	
___	___	___	9. Keep hands held upward to allow water to drip from the elbow. Dry with sterile towel.	

Name _Fallon Pryor_ Date _9/14/05_

Unit _____ Position _____

Instructor/Evaluator: _____ Position _____

Excellent	Satisfactory	Needs Practice	

PROCEDURE 26-3
APPLYING AND REMOVING STERILE GLOVES

Goal: To prevent transfer of microorganisms from hands to sterile objects or open wounds.

Comments

9/14
N Anderson RN MSN

APPLYING GLOVES

1. Wash hands.
2. Remove outside wrapper by peeling apart sides.
3. Lay inner package on clean, flat surface above waist level. Open wrapper from the outside, keeping gloves on inside surface.
4. Grasp inside edge of glove with thumb and first two fingers of dominant hand. Holding hands above waist, insert nondominant hand into glove. Adjust fingers inside glove after both gloves are on.
5. Slip gloved hand underneath second gloved cuff still in package, and pull over dominant hand.
6. Keeping hands above waist, adjust glove fit, touching only sterile areas.

REMOVING GLOVES

1. With dominant hand, grasp outer surface of nondominant glove just below thumb. Peel off without touching exposed wrist.
2. Place ungloved hand under thumb side of second cuff and peel off toward fingers, holding first glove inside second glove. Discard into appropriate receptacle.
3. Wash hands.

NA

Name _Fallon_   Date _____

Unit _____   Position _____

Instructor/Evaluator: _____   Position _____

PROCEDURE 26-4
DONNING A STERILE GOWN AND CLOSED GLOVING

Excellent	Satisfactory	Needs Practice	
			Goal: To apply attire necessary to carry out sterile procedures safely. **Comments**
	✓		1. Don all surgical attire (scrubs, shoe covers, cap or hood, face mask, and protective eye wear), and perform the surgical hand scrub as described in Procedure 26-2.
			Donning a Sterile Gown
			1. Grasp folded sterile gown at the neckline and step away from the sterile field. Allow gown to unfold gently, being careful that it does not touch the floor. The inside of the gown is toward the wearer.
			2. Holding the arms at shoulder level, grasp the sterile gown just below the neckband near the shoulders, and slide arms in the sleeves until the fingers are at the end of the cuffs but not through the cuffs.
	✓		3. Have someone tie the back of the gown, taking care that only the ties are touched and not the sides or front of the gown.
			Closed Gloving
	✓		1. With fingers still within the cuff of the gown, open the inner sterile glove package and pick up the first glove by the cuff using your nondominant hand.
			2. Position the glove over the cuff of the gown so the fingers are in alignment, and stretch the entire glove over the stockinet cuff, being careful not to touch the edge of the stockinet cuff. Fingers remain within the cuff of the gown.
			3. Work the fingers into the glove, and pull the glove up over the wrist with the nondominant hand that still remains within the cuff of the gown.
			4. Use the sterile gloved hand to pick up the second glove, placing it over the stockinet cuff of the dominant hand and repeating the glove application process.
	✓		5. Adjust gloves for comfort and fit, taking care to keep gloved hands above waist level at all times.

Comments: _(signature)_ 9/14/05

Name _____ Date _9/14/05_

Unit _____ Position _____

Instructor/Evaluator: _____ Position _____

Excellent	Satisfactory	Needs Practice	

PROCEDURE 26-5
PREPARING AND MAINTAINING A STERILE FIELD

Goal: To create an environment to prevent the transfer of microorganisms during sterile procedures.

Comments

1. Wash hands.
2. Inspect all sterile packages for package integrity, contamination, or moisture.
3. During entire procedure, never turn your back on the sterile field or lower your hands below the level of the field.

Opening a Sterile Drape

1. Remove the sterile drape from the outer wrapper, and place the inner drape in the center of the work surface at or above waist level with the outer flap facing away from you.
2. Touching the outside flap only, reach around (rather than over) the sterile field to open the flap away from you.
3. Open the side flaps in the same manner using the right hand for the right flap and the left hand for the left flap.
4. Open the innermost flap that faces you, being careful that it does not touch your clothing or any object.

Adding Sterile Supplies to the Field

1. Prepackaged sterile supplies are opened by peeling back the partially sealed edge with both hands or lifting up the unsealed edge taking care not to touch the supplies with your hands.
2. Hold supplies 10 to 12 inches above the field, allowing them to fall to the middle of the sterile field.
3. Grasp the corners of the wrapper with the free hand, and hold them against the wrist of the other hand while you carefully drip the object onto the sterile field.

Adding Solutions to a Sterile Field

1. Read the solution label and expiration date. Note any signs of contamination.
2. Remove cap and place it with the inside facing up on a flat surface. Do not touch inside of cap or rim of bottle.

PREPARING AND MAINTAINING A STERILE FIELD
(Continued)

Excellent	Satisfactory	Needs Practice		Comments
			3. Hold bottle 6 inches above container on the sterile field, and pour slowly to avoid spills.	
			4. Recap the solution bottle, and label it with date and time of opening if the solution is to be reused.	
			5. Add any additional supplies and don sterile gloves prior to starting the procedure.	

Name **Fallan Pryor** Date _____

Unit _____ Position _____

Instructor/Evaluator: _____ Position _____

Excellent	Satisfactory	Needs Practice	PROCEDURE 27-1 **ADMINISTERING ORAL MEDICATIONS**	Comments
			Goal: To provide a safe, effective, economic route for administering medications.	
			1. Wash hands.	
			2. Arrange MAR next to medication cart or cabinet, medication trays, and cups.	
			3. Prepare medications for only one client at a time.	
			4. Remove ordered medications from cart or shelf. Compare label on medication with MAR, and check the five rights of medication administration. Scan barcode if using Bar Code Medication Administration (BCMA). If a discrepancy exits, recheck the client's chart and medication orders.	
			5. Calculate correct drug dosage if necessary.	
			6. Prepare selected medications.	
			a. Unit dosage: Place packaged medications directly into medicine cup, or lay on tray without unwrapping.	
			b. Medications from a multidose bottle: Pour tablets or capsules into the container lid, and transfer into medicine cup. Return any extra tablets to the bottle.	
			c. Medications from a bingo card: Snap the bubble containing the correct medication directly over the medicine cup. Do not touch medications.	
			d. Swallowing difficulty: If client has trouble swallowing tablets, grind with mortar and pestle or other drug-crushing device until smooth. Mix powder in small amount of pudding or applesauce. Do not crush enteric-coated tablets or extended-release tablets.	
			e. Liquid medications: Remove cap and place on countertop inside up. Hold bottle so label is against palm of hand. Hold medication cup at eye level, and fill until bottom of meniscus is at desired dosage. Discard excess poured liquid from cup into sink. Do not pour back into bottle.	
			7. Take medication directly to client's room. Do not leave medication unattended.	

PROCEDURE 27-1
ADMINISTERING ORAL MEDICATIONS (Continued)

Excellent	Satisfactory	Needs Practice		Comments

Excellent · **Satisfactory** · **Needs Practice**

8. Compare name on MAR with name on client's identification band. If the client is not wearing an identification band, ask the client to state his or her name.

9. Complete any pre-administration assessment (i.e., blood pressure) the specific medication requires.

10. Compare medication to MAR, and recheck the five rights of medication administration. If using unit-dose medications, unwrap the medication and place in the cup before checking the five rights of the next medication.

11. Explain medication's purpose to client.

12. Assist client to sitting position if necessary. Give medication cup and glass of water to client.

13. If client is unable to hold the medication cup, place pill cup to lips and introduce medication into his or her mouth. If tablet or capsule falls on floor, discard and repeat preparation.

14. Stay with client until he or she swallows all medications. Look inside client's mouth if the client is cognitively impaired or has difficulty swallowing to ensure client receives the ordered medications.

15. Dispose of soiled supplies, and wash hands.

16. Record time medication was administered and any pre-administration assessment data collected.

Name ~~Fallon Pryor~~   Date ~~10/05~~

Unit _____   Position _____

Instructor/Evaluator: ~~G Swiney RN om~~   Position _____

Excellent	Satisfactory	Needs Practice	
			## PROCEDURE 27-2 ## ADMINISTERING MEDICATION ## BY METERED-DOSE INHALER

Goal: To deliver premeasured dose of medication to the bronchial airways and lungs.

Comments

Excellent	Satisfactory	Needs Practice	
10/05	—	—	1. Check medication order (see Procedure 27-1, Steps 1 to 5).
—	—	—	2. Assemble medication canister, inhalation mouthpiece, and spacer device if needed. Attach the medication canister to the inhaler mouthpiece by inserting the metal stem into the long end of the mouthpiece. Shake the canister several times.
—	—	—	3. Assist the client to sitting or standing position. Perform the second medication check of five rights.
—	—	—	4. Ask client to breathe out through his or her mouth.
—	—	—	5. Position the mouthpiece 1 to 2 inches from client's open mouth. Instruct the client to breathe in slowly through his or her mouth. As client starts inhaling, press the canister down to release one dose of the medication.
—	—	—	6. Instruct client to hold his or her breath for 10 seconds, if possible.
—	—	—	7. Wait at least 1 minute before administration of a second dose or inhalation of a different medication by MDI. Administer bronchodilators by MDI before other inhaled medications.
—	—	—	8. Wash hands and clean mouthpiece. If steroid medication was administered, have client rinse mouth.
—	—	—	9. Reassess ease of breathing, respiratory rate, accessory muscle use, and breath sounds.
—	—	—	10. Document medication administration and client status before and after administration.

Modification for Using a Spacer With an MDI

Excellent	Satisfactory	Needs Practice	
—	—	—	1. Attach spacer to inhalation mouthpiece. After exhaling, instruct client to place the mouthpiece in his or her mouth and close lips around the mouthpiece. Depress the medication canister and have client inhale. If client can't take and hold a deep breath, advise to take two or three short breaths to get all the medication from the spacer.

65

Name _____   Date _____

Unit _____   Position _____

Instructor/Evaluator: _____   Position _____

PROCEDURE 27-3
WITHDRAWING MEDICATION FROM A VIAL

Goal: To withdraw a precise amount of medication from a vial while maintaining asepsis.

Excellent	Satisfactory	Needs Practice		Comments

1. Check medication order, and compare the name of the ordered medication with the label on the medication vial (see Procedure 27-1, and complete Steps 1 to 5).
2. Assemble needle and syringe.
3. Pick up vial. If medication has been reconstituted or is in suspension, place vial between the palms, rotating or rolling the vial back and forth. Do not shake.
4. Remove metal cap from vial. Cleanse top of vial with alcohol wipe, and remove guard from needle.
5. Pull back on barrel of syringe to draw in a volume of air equal to the volume of the ordered medication dose. Holding vial between thumb and fingers of the nondominant hand, insert needle through the rubber stopper into the air space—not the solution—in the vial, and inject air.
6. Invert vial and withdraw the ordered dose of medication by pulling back on the plunger. Make sure needle is in the solution to be withdrawn.
7. Expel air bubbles and adjust dose if necessary.
8. Remove needle from vial, and cover the needle with guard.

Name _____   Date _____

Unit _____   Position _____

Instructor/Evaluator: _____   Position _____

Excellent	Satisfactory	Needs Practice	PROCEDURE 27-4 **WITHDRAWING MEDICATION FROM AN AMPULE**	Comments
			Goal: To withdraw full dose of medication from an ampule safely while maintaining asepsis.	
___	___	___	1. Check medication order, and make sure the solution in the ampule matches the ordered solution (see Procedure 27-1, and complete Steps 1 to 5).	
___	___	___	2. Assemble needle and syringe. Filter needle may be used.	
___	___	___	3. Pick up ampule and flick its upper stem several times with a fingernail.	
___	___	___	4. Wrap a sterile gauze pad or alcohol wipe around the neck of the ampule before breaking the neck with an outward snapping motion.	
___	___	___	5. Discard the broken neck appropriately, and prepare to withdraw medication from ampule using one of the following methods:	
___	___	___	a. Place ampule upright on a flat surface, insert needle in the solution, and withdraw the correct amount of medication by pulling up on the plunger without touching the needle to the glass rim.	
___	___	___	b. Invert the ampule or tilt it sideways. Insert the needle into the solution; pull back on the plunger, and withdraw the proper dose of medication.	
___	___	___	6. Remove needle from solution. Hold needle upright, inspect the syringe, and dispel any air that may have been drawn into the syringe. Make sure the syringe contains the correct amount of medication. Expel any extra medication into a container.	
___	___	___	7. Cover needle with guard, and change needle if filter needle was used. Discard ampule in sharps container.	
___	___	___	8. Wash hands.	

Name _____   Date _____

Unit _____   Position _____

Instructor/Evaluator: _____   Position _____

			PROCEDURE 27-5	
Excellent	**Satisfactory**	**Needs Practice**	# DRAWING UP TWO MEDICATIONS IN A SYRINGE	
			Goal: To minimize the number of injections a client receives and to prevent contaminating one vial of medication with medication from the other vial.	**Comments**
___	___	___	1. Wash hands.	
___	___	___	2. Compare medications to MAR (see Procedure 27-1, and complete Steps 1 to 5).	
___	___	___	3. Cleanse tops of both vials with antiseptic.	
___	___	___	4. With syringe, aspirate volume of air equal to medication dose from first medication (Vial A).	
___	___	___	5. Inject air into Vial A, being careful that needle does not touch solution.	
___	___	___	6. Remove syringe from Vial A. Aspirate volume of air equal to the medication dose from second medication (Vial B). Inject air into Vial B.	
___	___	___	7. Invert Vial B, and withdraw required volume of medication into syringe. Expel all air bubbles, and withdraw needle from Vial B.	
___	___	___	8. Determine what total combined volume of medication would measure on syringe scale.	
___	___	___	9. Insert needle into Vial A, invert vial, and carefully withdraw required volume of medication (as in Step 7).	
___	___	___	10. Withdraw needle from Vial A, and replace needle guard.	
___	___	___	11. Check medication and dosage before returning or discarding vials.	
			Modification for Insulin	
___	___	___	1. Wash hands.	
___	___	___	2. When preparing insulin in suspension, gently rotate vials between palms of hands to mix the suspension.	
___	___	___	3. Follow Steps 3 to 9 above.	
___	___	___	4. Establish routine order for drawing up insulin.	

Name _____ Date _____

Unit _____ Position _____

Instructor/Evaluator: _____ Position _____

Excellent	Satisfactory	Needs Practice	PROCEDURE 27-6 **ADMINISTERING INTRADERMAL INJECTIONS**	Comments
			Goal: To administer medication into dermal tissue to screen for allergic dermal reactions.	
___	___	___	1. Check medication order (see Procedure 27-1, Steps 1 to 5).	
___	___	___	2. Assemble needle and syringe.	
___	___	___	3. Remove needle guard, and withdraw medication from vial.	
___	___	___	4. Identify client by name or identification bracelet. Scan ID bracelet if using BCMA. Explain procedure to client. Repeat check of five rights.	
___	___	___	5. Select injection site that is relatively hairless and free from tenderness, swelling, scarring, or inflammation.	
___	___	___	6. Remove needle guard. Hold syringe in dominant hand. Gently pull skin distal to intended injection site taut with nondominant hand.	
___	___	___	7. Holding syringe from above, at a 10- to 15-degree angle (almost parallel to skin), gently insert needle, bevel up, until dermis barely covers bevel.	
___	___	___	8. Stabilize needle, then inject medication slowly over 3 to 5 seconds.	
___	___	___	9. Withdraw needle. Do **not** wipe or massage site.	
___	___	___	10. Do not recap needle. Dispose of syringe and needle in sharps container.	
___	___	___	11. Record time and site of injection according to agency protocol.	
___	___	___	12. Instruct client when to return for reading of response: 15 to 60 minutes after injection for allergy testing and usually 48 to 72 hours after injection for TST.	

Name _____   Date _____

Unit _____   Position _____

Instructor/Evaluator: _____   Position _____

Excellent	Satisfactory	Needs Practice	PROCEDURE 27-7 **ADMINISTERING SUBCUTANEOUS INJECTIONS**	Comments
			Goal: To ensure more rapid absorption and action of a medication than can be achieved orally.	
___	___	___	1. Check medication order (see Procedure 27-1, Steps 1 to 5).	
___	___	___	2. Assemble needle and syringe.	
___	___	___	3. Remove needle guard, and withdraw medication from container (see Procedures 27-3 and 27-4).	
___	___	___	4. Identify client by name or identification bracelet. Scan ID bracelet if using BCMA. Explain procedure to client. Recheck five rights.	
___	___	___	5. Don gloves.	
___	___	___	6. Select injection site that is free from tenderness, swelling, scarring, and inflammation.	
___	___	___	7. Cleanse site with antiseptic swab in circular motion from center outward. Allow area to dry thoroughly.	
___	___	___	8. Remove needle guard. Hold syringe in dominant hand. Place nondominant hand on either side of injection site. Spread or bunch skin to stabilize site and identify subcutaneous tissue.	
___	___	___	9. Hold syringe between thumb and forefinger of dominant hand. Inject needle quickly at a 45- to 90-degree angle, depending on amount of subcutaneous tissue. Release bunched skin.	
___	___	___	10. Aspirate by slowly pulling back on plunger. If blood appears in syringe, withdraw needle, discard syringe, and prepare a new injection.	
___	___	___	11. If no blood appears, inject medication with slow, even pressure.	
___	___	___	12. Remove needle quickly while pressing antiseptic swab over site.	
___	___	___	13. Gently massage site with antiseptic swab.	
___	___	___	14. Assist client to position of comfort.	
___	___	___	15. Do not recap needle. Dispose of syringe and needle in sharps container.	
___	___	___	16. Wash hands.	
___	___	___	17. Record according to agency protocol.	

PROCEDURE 27-7

ADMINISTERING SUBCUTANEOUS INJECTIONS
(Continued)

Excellent

Satisfactory

Needs Practice

Comments

Modification for Insulin Administration

1. Routine aspiration is not necessary.
2. Systematically rotate injection sites to prevent lipodystrophy and variable insulin absorption.
3. Instruct clients who self-administer insulin about not needing to cleanse site with alcohol before injection or to wear gloves.

Modification for Heparin Administration

1. The abdomen except for 1 to 2 inches on either side of umbilicus is most frequently used site.
2. Roll or gently bunch tissue between thumb and forefinger to ensure heparin is administered into subcutaneous tissue. Do not tightly pinch skin.
3. Because heparin is an anticoagulant, do not aspirate for blood return or massage skin after injection.
4. After injection, slowly and smoothly withdraw needle to prevent leakage into subcutaneous tissue.

Name _____   Date _____

Unit _____   Position _____

Instructor/Evaluator: _____   Position _____

Excellent	Satisfactory	Needs Practice	PROCEDURE 27-8 **ADMINISTERING INTRAMUSCULAR INJECTIONS** **Goal:** To administer medication deeply into muscle tissue, without injury to client.	Comments
___	___	___	1. Check medication order (see Procedure 27-1, Steps 1 to 5). Assemble needle and syringe.	
___	___	___	2. Prepare needle, syringe, and medication by following appropriate steps in Procedure 27-3 or Procedure 27-4.	
___	___	___	3. If medication is known to be irritating to subcutaneous tissues, replace needle after withdrawing medication.	
___	___	___	4. Identify client by name or identification bracelet. Scan ID bracelet if using BCMA. Explain procedure to client. Recheck five rights.	
___	___	___	5. Don gloves. Assist client to a comfortable position, and expose only the area to be injected.	
___	___	___	6. Select appropriate injection site by inspecting muscle size and integrity. Consider volume of medication to be injected. Use anatomic landmarks to locate exact injection site.	
___	___	___	7. Cleanse site with antiseptic swab, wiping from center of site and rotating outward. Remove needle guard. Hold syringe between thumb and forefinger of dominant hand (like a dart). Spread skin at the site with nondominant hand.	
___	___	___	8. Insert needle quickly at a 90-degree angle to client's skin surface.	
___	___	___	9. Stabilize syringe barrel by grasping with nondominant hand.	
___	___	___	a. Aspirate slowly by pulling back on plunger with dominant hand.	
___	___	___	b. If no blood appears, inject medication slowly.	
___	___	___	c. If blood appears in syringe, remove needle, dispose of syringe, and prepare new medication.	
___	___	___	10. Withdraw needle while pressing antiseptic swab above site.	
___	___	___	11. Gently massage site.	
___	___	___	12. Do not recap needle. Dispose of equipment in sharps container.	

Excellent	Satisfactory	Needs Practice	

PROCEDURE 27-8
ADMINISTERING INTRAMUSCULAR INJECTIONS(Continued)

Comments

___ ___ ___ 13. Wash hands.

___ ___ ___ 14. Record medication and client response according to agency protocol.

Variation for Air Lock Injection Technique

___ ___ ___ 1. Withdraw desired volume of medication into syringe.

___ ___ ___ 2. Draw in an additional 0.2 mL of air.

___ ___ ___ 3. Check medication dose in syringe; expel excess amount of medication from syringe.

___ ___ ___ 4. Redraw in 0.2 mL of air, and recheck dose accuracy.

___ ___ ___ 5. Insert the needle entering the client at a 90-degree angle to the client's skin surface and the floor. Position the client so the proper anatomic landmarks can be located for the chosen site and still allow the needle to enter the client at a 90-degree angle to the floor; for example, when using either the ventrogluteal or deltoid sites, the client must be side-lying.

Variation for Z-Track Injection

___ ___ ___ 1. When preparing injection site, pull skin and subcutaneous tissues about 1 to 1.5 inches to one side of the selected site.

___ ___ ___ 2. Insert syringe at a 90-degree angle.

___ ___ ___ 3. Aspirate and administer medication while continuing traction on skin.

___ ___ ___ 4. Leave needle inserted an additional 10 seconds.

___ ___ ___ 5. Simultaneously remove needle and release traction on skin.

Name _____   Date _____

Unit _____   Position _____

Instructor/Evaluator: _____   Position _____

Excellent	Satisfactory	Needs Practice	PROCEDURE 27-9 **ADMINISTERING MEDICATION BY INTRAVENOUS PUSH**	Comments
			Goal: To achieve high blood levels of a medication in a short time period.	
___	___	___	1. Check medication order (see Procedure 26-1, Steps 1 to 5).	
___	___	___	2. Recheck the five rights of medication administration.	
___	___	___	3. Prepare and draw up ordered medication from vial or ampule. Read package insert for proper amount and solution for dilution. Apply needleless adaptor or a small-gauge needle to syringe.	
___	___	___	4. Identify client by looking at nameband or asking name. Perform the third check of the five rights.	
___	___	___	5. Explain procedure to client.	
___	___	___	6. Don gloves.	
			Administering Medication Into an Existing Intravenous Line	
___	___	___	1. Select injection port in IV tubing closest to IV insertion site.	
___	___	___	2. If using a needle, cleanse injection port with antiseptic. Allow to dry.	
___	___	___	3. Insert needle into injection port or attach syringe to injection port (needleless system).	
___	___	___	4. Occlude the IV tubing above the injection port by pinching the tubing. Gently pull back on the syringe plunger until blood appears in the tubing.	
___	___	___	5. Inject medication slowly into the IV port at the prescribed rate. Use a watch to time administration rate.	
___	___	___	6. If IV medication and IV solution in tubing are incompatible, assess for blood return with 10 mL syringe of sterile normal saline solution.	
___	___	___	7. After confirming IV catheter placement, flush line with normal saline solution while occluding catheter above port.	
___	___	___	8. Administer medication at prescribed rate; reflush with 10 mL of sterile normal saline solution, and release occlusion.	
			Administering Medication Into Intermittent Injection Device or Lock Device	
___	___	___	1. Swab the injection port with antiseptic. Allow to dry.	

ADMINISTERING MEDICATION BY INTRAVENOUS PUSH (Continued)

Excellent	Satisfactory	Needs Practice		Comments
___	___	___	2. Attach syringe (needleless system) or insert needle of syringe with 1 mL normal saline solution into injection port. Gently pull back on syringe plunger to assess for blood return.	
___	___	___	3. Flush IV lock with 1 mL normal saline solution. Remove syringe.	
___	___	___	4. Attach syringe (needleless system) or insert needle of syringe with medication into injection port. Inject medication slowly at the prescribed rate. Use watch to time safe administration rate. Remove syringe.	
___	___	___	5. Attach syringe (needleless system) or insert needle of syringe with 1 to 3 mL of normal saline into injection port and flush the port with saline.	
___	___	___	6. Dispose of uncapped needles and syringes in sharps container.	
___	___	___	7. Wash hands.	
___	___	___	8. Document medication administration.	
___	___	___	9. Evaluate client's response to medication therapy.	

Name _____   Date _____

Unit _____   Position _____

Instructor/Evaluator: _____   Position _____

Excellent	Satisfactory	Needs Practice	PROCEDURE 27-10 **ADMINISTERING INTRAVENOUS MEDICATIONS USING INTERMITTENT INFUSION TECHNIQUE** **Goal:** To maintain therapeutic levels of medication in client's blood.	Comments
___	___	___	1. Check medication order (see Procedure 27-1, Steps 1 to 5).	
___	___	___	2. Prepare the medication syringe and IV tubing. Examine the syringe for any air bubbles, and expel any that are present. Attach the syringe to the extension tubing, and gently push the syringe plunger to prime tubing. Cover adaptor.	
___	___	___	3. Secure the medication syringe into the pump with the flange of the syringe in the clamp's groove.	
___	___	___	4. Confirm client's identity by looking at identification band or asking his or her name. Scan client's ID bracelet if using BCMA. Recheck the five rights, and explain the procedure to the client.	
___	___	___	5. Don gloves.	
___	___	___	6. Attach syringe with normal saline into the lock device. Flush lock with normal saline. Gently pull back on syringe plunger to assess for blood return.	
___	___	___	7. Attach tubing to lock device. Secure IV tubing to IV site with tape.	
___	___	___	8. Program the pump for the appropriate infusion speed and press the start key. The medication syringe label often indicates the suggested infusion speed, typically 30 to 60 minutes. If uncertain, consult a drug reference handbook or pharmacist.	
___	___	___	9. Document medication administration.	
___	___	___	10. Assess client and infusion device 5 to 10 minutes after infusion has begun.	
___	___	___	11. When the completion alarm sounds, return to client's room and press the pump's stop key.	
___	___	___	12. Don gloves. Remove tubing from lock device. Attach syringe with 1 to 3 mL normal saline or heparin flush solution and flush lock.	
___	___	___	13. Replace lock with new sterile cap.	
___	___	___	14. Dispose of syringes in proper container. Wash hands.	

Excellent

Satisfactory

Needs Practice

PROCEDURE 27-10
ADMINISTERING INTRAVENOUS MEDICATIONS USING INTERMITTENT INFUSION TECHNIQUE (Continued)

Comments

Variation Using Intravenous Bag and Gravity Intravenous Tubing

1. Check medication order (see Procedure 27-1, Steps 1 to 5).
2. Connect infusion tubing to medication bag (see Procedure 28-2).
3. Follow Steps 6 to 9 above.
4. Set IV drip rate to infuse medication over prescribed time. Monitor periodically.
5. Document medication administration.
6. When medication has infused, turn off flow clamp.
7. Follow Steps 14 to 17 above.

Variation When Administering Intermittent Intravenous Medication Into Primary Intravenous Line

1. Perform previous steps through second check of five rights.
2. Prepare medication, tubing, and pump, if used, according to procedures described above.
3. Confirm client's identity, and perform third medication check.
4. Hang syringe pump or medication bag at or above level of primary IV solution.
   a. If using a needle, wipe injection port nearest to the IV insertion site on primary IV tubing with antiseptic, and attach needle with needle protector.
   b. If using a needleless system, insert secondary line into the needleless adaptor port.
5. Check compatibility of medications to be administered with the IV solution being infused and any other infusing medications. If medications are not compatible with primary IV solution, clamp primary IV tubing above injection port, insert syringe with 20 mL of normal saline, flush solution, and flush IV line.
6. Secure secondary line (piggyback) to injection port or Y site on IV tubing closest to IV insertion site.
7. Start syringe pump or set drip rate.
8. When medication has infused, stop syringe pump or turn off flow clamp. Flush IV line with saline prn. Regulate primary infusion as necessary.

ADMINISTERING INTRAVENOUS MEDICATIONS USING INTERMITTENT INFUSION TECHNIQUE (Continued)

Excellent	Satisfactory	Needs Practice		Comments
⎯	⎯	⎯	9. Discard medication syringe or bag or reserve for next medication infusion. Follow agency guidelines.	
⎯	⎯	⎯	10. Wash hands.	
⎯	⎯	⎯	11. Document medication administration, and add IV volume to IV intake.	

Name _____   Date _____

Unit _____   Position _____

Instructor/Evaluator: _____   Position _____

Excellent	Satisfactory	Needs Practice	PROCEDURE 28-1 **MONITORING AN INTRAVENOUS INFUSION**	
			Goal: To provide a safe, patent route for infusion of IV fluid therapy.	**Comments**
___	___	___	1. Compare IV fluid currently infusing with the ordered solution.	
___	___	___	2. Inspect the rate of flow at least every hour. For gravity-regulated IVs, check actual flow rate for 15 seconds and compare with prescribed rate of flow. If infusion is ahead of schedule, slow it so the infusion will complete at the planned time. If infusion is behind schedule, review agency policy before increasing flow rate. Many agencies require a physician's order to increase the rate of flow. If electronic infusion device (EID) is used, the hourly infusion rate in milliliters per hour is programmed into the machine. Most EID manufacturers require use of cassette tubing unique to their machine.	
___	___	___	3. Inspect the system for leakage, and if present, locate the source. Tighten all connections within the system. If leak is still present, slow IV flow rate to keep vein open, and replace tubing with sterile set.	
___	___	___	4. Inspect the tubing for kinks or blockages. Loosely coil tubing and place it on the bed.	
___	___	___	5. Observe the fluid level in the drip chamber. If it is less than half full, squeeze the chamber gently to allow more fluid in.	
___	___	___	6. Inspect the infusion site for infiltration. This occurs when the needle becomes dislodged from the vein and IV fluid flows into the interstitial tissue. Look for signs of infiltration, including decreased rate of flow, swelling, pallor, coolness, and discomfort at or above the needle insertion site. If present, change the IV site. If a large amount of fluid infiltrated, elevate the arm above the heart on several pillows.	
___	___	___	7. Inspect arm above the insertion point for signs of phlebitis, including redness, swelling, warmth, and pain along the vein above the IV insertion site. If present, discontinue the IV and restart in another area.	

Excellent	Satisfactory	Needs Practice		Comments
——	——	——	8. Inspect the insertion site for bleeding.	
——	——	——	9. Although monitoring IV therapy is a nursing responsibility, if client is able to comply, teach to contact the nurse if the following occur:	
——	——	——	a. The flow rate changes suddenly.	
——	——	——	b. The fluid container is almost empty.	
——	——	——	c. Blood is in the tubing.	
——	——	——	d. The site becomes uncomfortable.	
——	——	——	10. Chart any findings indicating complications of IV therapy (e.g., infiltration).	

Name _____   Date _____

Unit _____   Position _____

Instructor/Evaluator: _____   Position _____

Excellent	Satisfactory	Needs Practice	PROCEDURE 28-2 **CHANGING INTRAVENOUS SOLUTION AND TUBING**	Comments
			Goal: To deliver IV therapy as ordered and decrease risk of client infection.	
			Changing Solution Container	
___	___	___	1. Wash hands.	
___	___	___	2. Compare solution with physician's order. Adhere to five rights of medication administration.	
___	___	___	3. Remove IV bag from outer wrapper. Look for leaks or impurities in the bag.	
___	___	___	4. Label solution container with client's name, solution type, additives, date, and time hung. Check prelabeled container with physician's order. Line up time strip with volume amount on bag or bottle. Record solution change in the client's record.	
			5. Prepare container for spiking:	
___	___	___	a. If solution is in a plastic bag, remove plastic cover from entry nipple. Maintain sterility of nipple end.	
___	___	___	b. If solution is in a bottle, remove metal cap, metal disk, and rubber disk. Maintain sterility of bottle top.	
___	___	___	6. Close clamp on the existing tubing.	
___	___	___	7. Take old solution container from pole and invert it.	
___	___	___	8. Remove spike from used container, maintaining its sterility. Spike new IV container with firm push/twist motion.	
___	___	___	9. Hang new container on IV pole.	
___	___	___	10. Inspect tubing for air bubbles, and assess that drip chamber is one half full of solution.	
___	___	___	11. Adjust clamp to regulate flow rate or program EID, according to orders.	
			Changing Solution and Tubing	
___	___	___	1. Follow only first three steps of Changing Solution Container.	
___	___	___	2. Open new tubing package, keeping protective covers on spike and catheter adapter.	

PROCEDURE 28-2
CHANGING INTRAVENOUS SOLUTION AND TUBING
(Continued)

Excellent Satisfactory Needs Practice

Comments

3. Adjust roller clamp on new tubing to fully closed position.

4. Prepare new solution container as directed in Step 5 of Changing Solution Container.

5. Remove protective cover from spike, maintaining sterility, and spike into new solution container.

6. Hang container and "prime" drip chamber by squeezing gently, allowing to fill one-half full.

7. Remove protective cap from catheter adapter, and adjust roller clamp to flush tubing with fluid. Replace protective cap.

8. Adjust roller clamp on old tubing to close fully.

9. Place towel or disposable underpad under extremity. Don clean, disposable gloves.

10. Hold catheter hub with fingers of one hand (may use hemostat). With other hand, loosen tubing using gentle twisting motion. Remove old dressings if necessary.

11. Grasp new tubing, remove protective catheter cap, and insert tightly into needle hub, while continuing to stabilize catheter hub with the other hand.

12. Adjust roller clamp to start solution flowing according to physician's order.

13. Remove and discard gloves.

14. Secure tubing with tape.

15. If dressing was removed, apply new dressing to IV site according to agency policy.

16. Label new tubing with date, time, and your initials.

17. Label solution container with client's name, solution type, additives, date, and time hung. Time label side of container.

18. Record solution and tubing change.

Name _____ Date _____

Unit _____ Position _____

Instructor/Evaluator: _____ Position _____

Excellent	Satisfactory	Needs Practice	PROCEDURE 28-3

PROCEDURE 28-3
CONVERTING TO AN INTERMITTENT INFUSION DEVICE (IID) AND FLUSHING

Goal: To maintain patency of intermittently used IV access.

Comments

Excellent	Satisfactory	Needs Practice	
___	___	___	1. Wash hands.
___	___	___	2. Explain procedure to client.
___	___	___	3. Prepare syringe with heparin flush solution or saline solution according to agency policy and manufacturer's recommendations for the type of device in place (may use between 0.5 and 1 mL [peripheral], 2.5 and 3 mL [central line] heparin flush, or 1 and 3 mL normal saline). Note: If flushing lock after administering a prescribed medication, a saline flush may be required, followed by a heparin flush to clear the medication completely from the catheter to prevent incompatibilities with heparin.
___	___	___	4. Obtain appropriate IID.
___	___	___	5. Don clean gloves.

Converting IV to an Intermittent Infusion Device

Excellent	Satisfactory	Needs Practice	
___	___	___	1. Clamp tubing of IV infusion with roller clamp.
___	___	___	2. Hold the catheter hub firmly with your nondominant hand (a hemostat may be used if necessary). With dominant hand, quickly twist IV tubing to the left to loosen but not disconnect from IV catheter.
___	___	___	3. Take IID out of package, keeping tip sterile. Hold in dominant hand between thumb and finger.
___	___	___	4. Stabilize IV catheter with nondominant hand as you disconnect IV tubing. Quickly insert IID into IV catheter, twisting to the right to tighten.
___	___	___	5. Tape IID to stabilize. Redress using transparent dressing if necessary.

Flushing With Needle Type System

Excellent	Satisfactory	Needs Practice	
___	___	___	1. Perform Steps 1 to 5 above.
___	___	___	2. Swab injection port with antiseptic swab and allow to dry.
___	___	___	3. Insert needleless syringe into the port, and aspirate gently for evidence of blood return.

CONVERTING TO AN INTERMITTENT INFUSION DEVICE (IID) AND FLUSHING (Continued)

Excellent	Satisfactory	Needs Practice		Comments
___	___	___	4. Inject the recommended amount of saline or heparin flush, ending with 0.5 mL of solution remaining in syringe.	
___	___	___	5. Dispose of uncapped needles and syringes in proper container.	
___	___	___	6. Wash hands.	
___	___	___	7. Document date, time, route, amount, and type of flush solution. Also document assessment of site.	

Name _____   Date _____

Unit _____   Position _____

Instructor/Evaluator: _____   Position _____

Excellent	Satisfactory	Needs Practice	PROCEDURE 28-4 **ADMINISTERING TOTAL PARENTERAL NUTRITION (TPN)**	
			Goal: To provide parenteral nutritional support to selected clients.	**Comments**
			Monitoring Total Parenteral Nutrition Therapy	
___	___	___	1. Schedule and assist client with chest x-ray after central catheter insertion.	
___	___	___	2. Confirm correct solution is running at ordered rate. Check expiration date of solution. Use infusion controller to monitor and regulate flow rate. Infuse solutions with 10% dextrose or more directly into subclavian or internal jugular vein to dilute the solution rapidly and prevent thrombophlebitis.	
___	___	___	3. Inspect tubing and catheter connection for leaks or kinks. Tape all connections. Change tubing every 24 hours according to agency policy.	
___	___	___	4. Inspect insertion site for infiltration, thrombophlebitis, or drainage. If present, notify physician.	
___	___	___	5. Monitor vital signs, including temperature, every 4 hours.	
___	___	___	6. Assess for symptoms of air embolism: decreased level of consciousness, tachycardia, dyspnea, anxiety, "feeling of impending doom," chest pain, cyanosis, hypotension. If suspected, lay client on left side with head in Trendelenburg position.	
___	___	___	7. Use TPN line *only* for TPN and lipids. Never use for any other reason.	
___	___	___	8. Perform test for glucose every 6 hours. Notify physician if abnormal.	
___	___	___	9. Monitor laboratory tests of electrolytes, BUN, and glucose, as ordered, and report abnormal findings.	
___	___	___	10. Maintain accurate record of intake and output to monitor fluid balance.	
___	___	___	11. Weigh client daily and record.	
___	___	___	12. Inspect dressing once a shift for drainage and intactness. Change whenever loose or moist and at least every 48 hours.	

ADMINISTERING TOTAL PARENTERAL NUTRITION (TPN)
(Continued)

Excellent	Satisfactory	Needs Practice		Comments

Administering Intralipids

1. Check solution against physician's order. Inspect solution for separation of emulsion into layers or for froth. Do not use if present.

2. Wash hands.

3. Attach fat emulsion tubing to bottle. Prime tubing as for conventional IV.

4. Identify client.

5. Identify Y-port on hyperalimentation tubing (below in-line filter).

6. Cleanse Y-port with antiseptic swab. Allow to dry. Insert connector into port. Secure with tape. *Note:* Lipids can be infused into a peripheral IV.

7. Adjust flow rate to infuse at 1 mL/min for adults and 0.1 mL/min for children. Infuse at this rate for 30 minutes while monitoring the client and vital signs every 10 minutes. Note: If any adverse reactions occur, stop infusion and notify physician.

8. If no adverse reactions occur, adjust flow rate:

   a. Adults: 500 mL intralipid over 4 to 6 hours.

   b. Children: up to 1 g/kg over 4 hours.

9. Document procedure according to agency policy.

Name _____ Date _____

Unit _____ Position _____

Instructor/Evaluator: _____ Position _____

Excellent	Satisfactory	Needs Practice	PROCEDURE 28-5 **ADMINISTERING A BLOOD TRANSFUSION**	
			Goal: To replace blood volume or blood components lost through trauma, surgery, or a disease process.	**Comments**
——	——	——	1. Explain procedure to client. Have client sign consent form if required by agency policy.	
——	——	——	2. Obtain client's vital signs, including temperature.	
——	——	——	3. With another RN at client's bedside, verify the blood product and the client's identity by comparing the laboratory blood record with the following:	
——	——	——	a. Client's name and identification number both verbally and against client's wrist band.	
——	——	——	b. Blood unit number on the blood bag label.	
——	——	——	c. Blood group and RH type on the blood bag label.	
——	——	——	d. Verify the type of blood component and the expiration date noted on the blood label.	
——	——	——	e. Document verification by both RN signatures on transfusion record.	
——	——	——	4. Wash hands.	
——	——	——	5. Open Y-type blood administration set, and clamp both rollers completely.	
——	——	——	6. Spike 0.9% NaCl container. Prime drip chamber and tubing with saline.	
——	——	——	7. Spike blood or blood component unit with second spike. Keep roller clamp shut.	
——	——	——	8. Remove primary IV tubing from catheter hub, and cover end with sterile protector.	
——	——	——	9. Attach blood administration tubing to catheter hub and secure with tape.	
——	——	——	10. Flush line with NS. Open clamp to blood product. Open roller clamp below drip chamber and begin transfusion.	
——	——	——	11. Infuse blood slowly for first 15 minutes at 10 drops per minute.	
——	——	——	12. Monitor and document vital signs every 5 minutes during first 15 minutes, assessing for chilling, back pain, headache, nausea or vomiting, tachycardia, hypotension, tachypnea, or skin rash.	

Excellent	Satisfactory	Needs Practice		Comments
——	——	——	13. If any adverse reactions occur, close clamp to blood, open clamp to 0.9% NaCl, and notify physician immediately. Follow agency policy for laboratory notification and obtaining blood and urine specimens.	
——	——	——	14. If no adverse reactions occur after 15 minutes, regulate clamp to increase infusion according to physician's order. A unit of blood is usually administered over 2 hours. Monitor vital signs hourly until transfusion is complete.	
——	——	——	15. When blood transfusion is complete, clamp roller to blood and open roller to 0.9% NaCl solution. Infuse until tubing is clear.	
——	——	——	16. Obtain and document post-transfusion vital signs.	
——	——	——	17. If second blood component unit is to be transfused, slow 0.9% NaCl solution to keep vein open until next unit is available. Follow verification procedure and vital sign monitoring for each unit.	
——	——	——	18. If transfusion orders are complete, disconnect the blood administration tubing from catheter hub. Reconnect primary intravenous solution and tubing and adjust to desired rate.	
——	——	——	19. Wash hands.	
——	——	——	20. Document procedure on client's record.	

Name _____ Date _____

Unit _____ Position _____

Instructor/Evaluator: _____ Position _____

Excellent	Satisfactory	Needs Practice	PROCEDURE 32-1 **ASSISTING WITH THE BATH OR SHOWER**	Comments
			Goal: To cleanse the skin, stimulate circulation, control body odors, and promote self-esteem.	
___	___	___	1. Make sure tub and shower are clean.	
___	___	___	2. Place towel or disposable bath mat on floor by tub or shower.	
___	___	___	3. Accompany or transport client to bathroom. Use shower chair, if indicated.	
___	___	___	4. Place "occupied" sign on bathroom door.	
___	___	___	5. Keep client covered with bath blanket until water is ready.	
___	___	___	6. Fill bathtub halfway with warm water (105° F). Test water or have client test water. If client is taking shower, turn shower on and adjust temperature.	
___	___	___	7. Help client into shower or tub, providing necessary assistance.	
___	___	___	8. Instruct client to use safety bars and call bell signal. Client may prefer to sit in shower chair to prevent fatigue.	
___	___	___	9. If client is unable to shower independently, stay with client at all times. Use handheld shower to wash client.	
___	___	___	10. If client is showering or bathing independently, check on client within 15 minutes. Wash any areas he or she could not reach.	
___	___	___	11. Help client out of tub or shower. Assist with drying. If client is unsteady, drain water before getting client out of tub to prevent falls.	
___	___	___	12. Assist client with dressing and grooming.	
___	___	___	13. Help client to room. Return to bathroom to clean tub or shower according to agency policy. Discard soiled linen. Place "unoccupied" sign on door.	

Name Fallan Pryor   Date 9/7/05

Unit _____   Position _____

Instructor/Evaluator: _____   Position _____

PROCEDURE 32-2
BATHING A CLIENT IN BED

Goal: To cleanse the skin, stimulate circulation, control body odors, and promote self-esteem.

Excellent	Satisfactory	Needs Practice		Comments

1. Close curtains around bed or shut room door.
2. Help client to use bedpan, urinal, or commode, if needed.
3. Close window and doors to decrease drafts.
4. Wash your hands.
5. Raise bed to high position. Lock side rail up on opposite side of bed from your work.
6. Remove top sheet and bed spread, and place bath blanket on client. Help client move closer to you, and remove gown. If client has an IV line, remove gown from arm, lower IV container, and slide it through gown with tubing. Rehang IV container and check flow rate. Note: If reusing top linen, place it on back of chair; otherwise, place in laundry bag.
7. Lay towel across client's chest.
8. Wet washcloth and fold around your finger to make a mitt.
   a. Fold washcloth in thirds.
   b. Straighten washcloth to take out wrinkles.
   c. Fold washcloth over to fit hand.
   d. Tuck loose ends under edge of washcloth on palm.
9. Cleanse eyes with water only, wiping from inner to outer canthus. Use separate corner of mitt for each eye.
10. Determine if client would like soap used on face. Wash face, neck, and ears. Avoid letting soap sit in washbasin, or water will become too soapy for rinse. Liquid nondetergent cleansing agents, used in many agencies, do not require rinsing.
11. Fold bath blanket off arm away from you. Place towel lengthwise under arm. Wash, rinse, and dry the arm using long firm strokes from fingers toward axilla. Wash axilla.
12. (Optional) Place bath towel on bed and put wash basin on it. Immerse client's hand and allow to soak for several minutes. Wash, rinse, and dry hand well. Repeat on other side. Apply lotion.

PROCEDURE 32-2
BATHING A CLIENT IN BED (Continued)

Excellent	Satisfactory	Needs Practice		Comments

13. Repeat for arm and hand nearest you.

14. Apply deodorant or powder according to client's preferences. Avoid excessive use of powder or inhalation of powder.

15. Assess temperature of bath water, and change water if necessary. If you leave bedside, raise side rails to prevent accidental falls.

16. Place bath towel over chest. Fold bath blanket down to below umbilicus.

17. Lift bath towel off chest, and bathe chest and abdomen with mitted hand using long, firm strokes. Give special attention to skin under breasts and any other skin folds if client is overweight. Rinse and dry well.

18. Help client don clean gown.

19. Expose leg away from you by folding over bath blanket. Be careful to keep perineum covered.

20. Lift leg and place bath towel lengthwise under leg. Wash, rinse, and dry leg using long, firm strokes from ankle to thigh.

21. Wash feet or place in basin of water as for hands. Rinse and dry well. Pay special attention to space between toes.

22. Repeat for other leg and foot.

23. Assess bath water for warmth. Change water if necessary.

24. Assist client to side-lying position. Place bath towel along side of back and buttocks to protect linen. Wash, rinse, and dry back and buttocks. Give backrub with powder or lotion.

25. Assist to supine position. Assess if client can wash genitals and perineal area independently. If unable to, drape with bath blanket so that only genitals are exposed. Don disposable, clean gloves; using fresh water and a new cloth, wash, rinse, and dry genitalia and perineum.

26. Apply powder, lotion, cologne according to client preference.

27. Assist with hair and mouth care.

28. Make bed with clean linen.

29. Clean equipment and return to appropriate storage area.

30. Wash your hands.

31. Chart significant observations.

Name _____Fuller_____ Date _____

Unit _____ Position _____

Instructor/Evaluator: _____ Position _____

Excellent	Satisfactory	Needs Practice	

PROCEDURE 32-3
MASSAGING THE BACK

Goal: To stimulate circulation to the skin and promote comfort and relaxation.

Comments

1. Help client to side-lying or prone position.
2. Expose back, shoulders, upper arms, and sacral area. Cover remainder of body with bath blanket.
3. Wash hands in warm water. Warm lotion by holding container under running warm water.
4. Pour small amount of lotion into palms.
5. Begin massage in sacral area with circular motion. Move hands upward to shoulders, massaging over scapulae in smooth, firm strokes. Without removing hands from skin, continue in smooth strokes to upper arms and down sides of back to iliac crest. Continue for 3 to 5 minutes.
6. While massaging, assess for whitish or reddened areas that do not disappear and broken skin areas. Avoid pressure over areas of breakdown or redness.
7. If additional stimulation is desired, pétrissage (kneading) over shoulders and gluteal area and tapotement (tapping) up and down spine can be done.
8. End massage with long, continuous, stroking movements.
9. Pat excess lubricant dry with towel. Retie gown and assist to comfortable position.
10. Wash hands.

Name _____ Geller _____ Date _____

Unit _____ Position _____

Instructor/Evaluator: _____ Position _____

Excellent	Satisfactory	Needs Practice	PROCEDURE 32-4 **PERFORMING FOOT AND NAIL CARE**	Comments
			Goal: To maintain skin integrity around nails and maintain foot function.	
—	—	—	1. Wash hands.	2/ day 7 sept 05
—	—	—	2. Identify client. Help to chair if possible. Elevate head of bed for bedridden client.	
—	—	—	3. Fill washbasin with warm water (100°–104° F). Place waterproof pad under basin. Soak client's hands or feet in basin. Diabetic clients should *not* soak feet.	
—	—	—	4. Place call bell within reach. Allow hands or feet to soak for 10 to 20 minutes.	
—	—	—	5. Dry hand or foot that has been soaking. Rewarm water and allow other extremity to soak while you work on the softened nails.	
—	—	—	6. Gently clean under nails with orange stick. If nails are thickened and yellow, client may have fungal infection. Don disposable, clean gloves.	
—	—	—	7. Beginning with large toe or thumb, clip nail straight across. Shape nail with file. File rather than cut nails of clients with diabetes or circulatory problems.	
—	—	—	8. Push cuticle back gently with orange stick.	
—	—	—	9. Repeat procedure with other nails.	
—	—	—	10. Rinse foot or hand in warm water.	
—	—	—	11. Dry thoroughly with towel, especially between digits.	
—	—	—	12. Apply lotion to hands or feet.	
—	—	—	13. Help client to comfortable position.	
—	—	—	14. Remove and dispose of equipment.	
—	—	—	15. Wash hands.	

Name _____ *Fuller* _____ Date _____

Unit _____ Position _____

Instructor/Evaluator: _____ Position _____

Excellent	Satisfactory	Needs Practice	PROCEDURE 32-5 **SHAMPOOING HAIR OF A BEDRIDDEN CLIENT**	Comments
			Goal: To cleanse hair and scalp.	
—	—	—	1. Place waterproof pads under client's head and shoulders and remove pillow.	
—	—	—	2. Raise bed to highest position.	
—	—	—	3. Remove any pins from hair. Comb and brush hair thoroughly.	
—	—	—	4. Adjust bed to flat position. Place shampooing basin under head. Place bath towel around shoulders and folded washcloth where neck rests on basin.	
—	—	—	5. Fold bed linens down to waist. Cover upper body with bath blanket.	
—	—	—	6. Place waste basket with plastic bag under spout of shampoo basin on a chair or table at the bedside.	
—	—	—	7. Using water pitcher, wet hair thoroughly with warm water (approximately 110°F). Check temperature by placing small amount of water on your wrist.	
—	—	—	8. Apply small amount of shampoo. If needed, use hydrogen peroxide to dissolve matted blood in hair. Reassure client it will not bleach the hair.	
—	—	—	9. Massage scalp with fingertips while making shampoo lather. Start at hairline and work toward neck.	
—	—	—	10. Rinse hair with warm water. Reapply shampoo and repeat massage.	
—	—	—	11. Rinse hair thoroughly with warm water.	
—	—	—	12. Apply small amount of conditioner per client request. Rinse well.	
—	—	—	13. Squeeze excess moisture from hair. Wrap bath towel around hair. Rub to dry hair and scalp. Use second towel if necessary.	
—	—	—	14. Remove equipment and wet towels from bed. Place dry towel around client's shoulders.	
—	—	—	15. Dry hair with hair dryer. Comb and style.	
—	—	—	16. Help client to comfortable position.	
—	—	—	17. Dispose of soiled equipment and linen.	

Name _____   Date _____

Unit _____   Position _____

Instructor/Evaluator: _____   Position _____

PROCEDURE 32-6
PROVIDING ORAL CARE

Excellent	Satisfactory	Needs Practice	**Goal:** To cleanse tooth and mouth surfaces to prevent odor and caries.	Comments
—	—	—	1. Wash hands.	
—	—	—	2. Close bedside curtains or room door, identify client, and explain procedure.	
—	—	—	3. Help client to a sitting position. If client cannot sit, help to a side-lying position.	
—	—	—	4. Place towel under client's chin.	
—	—	—	5. Moisten toothbrush with water. Apply small amount of toothpaste.	
—	—	—	6. Hand toothbrush to client, or don disposable gloves and brush client's teeth as follows:	
—	—	—	a. Hold toothbrush at a 45-degree angle to gum line.	
—	—	—	b. Using short, vibrating motions, brush from gum line to crown of each tooth. Repeat until outside and inside of teeth and gums are cleaned.	
—	—	—	c. Cleanse biting surfaces by brushing with back and forth stroke.	
—	—	—	d. Brush tongue lightly. Avoid stimulating the gag reflex.	
—	—	—	7. Have client rinse mouth thoroughly with water and spit into emesis basin.	
—	—	—	8. Remove emesis basin, set aside, and dry client's mouth with washcloth.	
—	—	—	9. Floss client's teeth.	
—	—	—	a. Cut 10-inch piece of dental floss. Wind ends of floss around middle finger of each hand.	
—	—	—	b. Using index fingers to stretch the floss, move the floss up and down around and between lower teeth. Start at the back lower teeth and work around to other side.	
—	—	—	c. Using thumb and index fingers to stretch floss, repeat procedure on upper teeth.	
—	—	—	d. Have client rinse mouth thoroughly and spit into emesis basin.	
—	—	—	10. Remove basin. Dry client's mouth.	

PROCEDURE 32-6

PROVIDING ORAL CARE (Continued)

Excellent	Satisfactory	Needs Practice		Comments

11. Remove and dispose of supplies. Help client to comfortable position.

12. Wash hands.

Variations for the Unconscious Client

1. Gather equipment.

2. Place client in a side-lying position.

3. Place towel or waterproof pad under client's chin.

4. Place emesis basin against client's mouth, or have suction catheter positioned to remove secretions from mouth.

5. Use padded tongue blade to open teeth gently. Leave in place between the back molars. Never put your fingers in an unconscious client's mouth.

6. Brush teeth and gums as directed previously, using toothbrush or soft sponge-ended swab.

7. Swab or suction to remove pooled secretions. A small bulb syringe or syringe without needle may be used to rinse oral cavity.

8. Apply thin layer of petroleum jelly to lips to prevent drying or cracking. Note: Lemon and glycerine swabs can be drying to oral mucosa if used for extended periods.

Name _Jullen Roya_   Date _9/7/05_

Unit _____   Position _____

Instructor/Evaluator: _____   Position _____

Excellent	Satisfactory	Needs Practice		Comments

PROCEDURE 32-7
USING A BEDPAN

Goal: To provide a means for elimination for clients who are confined to bed or unable to get to the bathroom or bedside commode.

Placing the Bedpan

1. Wash hands. Don clean gloves.
2. Close curtain around bed or shut door.
3. Run warm water over rim of pan; dry with towel.
4. Position and lock side rail up on opposite side of bed from which you work.
5. Raise bed to height appropriate for nurse.
6. If client can raise buttocks and assist:
   a. Fold top linen down on nurse's side to expose client's hips.
   b. Have client flex knees and lift buttocks. Assist by placing your hand under sacrum, elbow on mattress, and lifting as a lever.
   c. Slide rounded smooth rim of regular bedpan under client. If using fracture pan, slide narrow flat end under buttocks.
7. For client unable to assist by raising buttocks:
   a. Lower head of bed to flat position.
   b. Fold top linens down to expose client minimally.
   c. Help client roll to side-lying position.
   d. Place bedpan against buttocks and tucked down against mattress. Hold firmly in place and roll client onto back as bedpan positions under buttocks.
8. Cover client with linen. Place call bell and toilet paper within reach.
9. Raise head of bed 45 to 80 degrees unless contraindicated.
10. Lower bed to lowest position. Place side rails up if indicated.
11. Remove gloves. Wash hands. Allow client to be alone.

PROCEDURE 32-7
USING A BEDPAN (Continued)

Excellent	Satisfactory	Needs Practice		Comments

Removing the Bedpan

12. Answer call bell promptly.

13. Place soap, wet washcloth, and towel at bedside.

14. Raise bed to appropriate working height for nurse.

15. Fold back top linens to expose client minimally.

16. Put on disposable clean gloves.

17. Assess if client can wipe perineal area. If not, wipe area with several layers of toilet tissue. If specimen is to be measured or collected, dispose of soiled toilet tissue in separate receptacle, not bedpan. (For female clients, wipe from urethra to anus.)

18. For client who can raise buttocks and assist with procedure:

    a. Lower head of bed.

    b. Have client flex knees and lift buttocks. Assist by placing one hand under sacrum and supporting bedpan with other hand to prevent spillage. Remove bedpan and place on bedside chair.

    c. Offer soap, warm water, washcloth, and towel for client to wash hands or perineal area.

19. For client unable to assist by raising buttocks:

    a. Lower head of bed to flat position.

    b. Fold top linen down to expose client minimally.

    c. Help client to roll off bedpan and onto side. Use one hand to stabilize bedpan during turning to prevent spillage.

    d. Wipe anal area with tissue. Wash perineum with soap and warm water. Pat dry.

20. Assist client to comfortable position.

21. Cover bedpan and remove from bedside. Obtain specimen if required. Empty and clean bedpan and return it to bedside.

22. Remove and discard gloves. Wash hands.

23. Spray air freshener if necessary to control odor, unless contraindicated (respiratory conditions, allergies).

Comments (handwritten): N Anderson RN MSN 9/7

Name _Fallan Pryor_   Date _9/7/05_

Unit _____   Position _____

Instructor/Evaluator: _____   Position _____

Excellent	Satisfactory	Needs Practice	PROCEDURE 32-8 **MAKING AN UNOCCUPIED BED**	Comments
			Goal: To provide clean linen and remove sources of skin irritation.	
___	___	___	1. Wash hands. Assemble equipment on bedside table or chair.	
___	___	___	2. Help client to chair at bedside.	
___	___	___	3. Raise bed to comfortable working position.	
___	___	___	4. Loosen linen on one side of bed. Move to other side of bed, and loosen all linen.	
___	___	___	5. Remove bedspread and blanket and fold each separately if they are to be reused. Place over back of chair.	
___	___	___	6. Remove pillowcases by grasping seamed end with one hand and pulling pillow out with the other. Place pillows on chair. Discard pillowcases in linen bag.	
___	___	___	7. Remove each piece of linen separately by rolling into a ball and discarding into linen bag. Be careful to prevent soiled linen from touching your uniform.	
___	___	___	8. Slide mattress to head of bed if it has slipped to the foot. Wipe mattress with antiseptic solution if grossly soiled. Dry thoroughly.	
___	___	___	9. Working from side of bed where linen is stored, spread mattress pad over mattress and smooth out wrinkles.	
___	___	___	10. Unfold bottom sheet lengthwise on bed with vertical center crease along center of bed. Unfold top layer toward opposite side of mattress. Pull remaining top sheet over head of mattress, leaving bottom edge of sheet even with mattress edge. Smooth bottom sheet with hand.	
___	___	___	11. Standing near head of bed, tuck excess sheet under the mattress on your side at the end of the bed.	
___	___	___	12. Miter the corner on your side:	
___	___	___	a. Grasp side edge of sheet about 18 inches down from mattress top.	
___	___	___	b. Lay sheet on top of mattress to form triangular, flat fold.	
___	___	___	c. Tuck sheet hanging loose below mattress under the mattress, without pulling on triangular fold.	
___	___	___	d. Pick up top of triangular fold and place it over side of mattress.	

PROCEDURE 32-8
MAKING AN UNOCCUPIED BED (Continued)

Excellent	Satisfactory	Needs Practice		Comments

e. Tuck this loose portion of sheet under mattress. Tuck remaining sheet on that side under the mattress. Lay draw sheet, folded in half, on the bed with the center fold at center of bed. Place top edge of draw sheet about 12 to 15 inches from head of bed. Tuck excess draw sheet under mattress.

13. Move to opposite side of bed.

14. Spread bottom sheet over mattress edge and miter top corner.

15. Tuck excess bottom sheet tightly under mattress, pulling gently to smooth out wrinkles.

16. Grasp draw sheet, pulling gently. Beginning at middle, tuck draw sheet under mattress firmly. Finish tucking top and bottom.

17. Return to side of bed where linen is placed.

18. Place top sheet on bed with vertical center fold at center of bed. Unfold sheet with seams facing out and top edge even with top of mattress. Smooth sheet, with excess falling over bottom edge of mattress.

19. Spread blanket and bedspread evenly over bed. Miter the bottom corner, using all three layers of linen (sheet, blanket, bedspread). Leave sides untucked.

20. Move to opposite side of bed and miter bottom corner, using all three linen layers.

21. Standing at bottom of bed, grasp top covers about 10 inches from bottom of mattress. Loosen linen slightly by pulling on top covers or forming a pleat.

22. Put on clean pillowcases:

  a. Grasp center of pillowcase, with one hand on seamed end.

  b. Gather case, turning it inside out over the hand holding it.

  c. With same hand, grasp middle of one end of pillow.

  d. Pull case over pillow with free hand.

  e. Adjust case so corners fit over pillow.

23. Place pillows in center at head of bed.

24. Fold top linen back to one side or fanfold at bottom of bed.

PROCEDURE 32-8
MAKING AN UNOCCUPIED BED (Continued)

Excellent	Satisfactory	Needs Practice		Comments
—	⟩	—	25. Secure call bell within client's reach and lower bed.	
—		—	26. Arrange bedside table, nightstand, and personal items within easy reach.	
—	✓	—	27. Discard soiled linen according to agency policy.	
—		—	28. Wash hands.	

Name _Fallan Bryd_   Date _9/7/0_

Unit _____   Position _____

Instructor/Evaluator: _____   Position _____

PROCEDURE 32-9
MAKING AN OCCUPIED BED

Excellent	Satisfactory	Needs Practice		Comments
			Goal: To provide clean linen for client who is unable to get out of bed	
—	—	—	1. Wash hands.	
—	—	—	2. Assemble equipment on bedside table or chair.	
—	—	—	3. Close door or bedside curtains.	
—	—	—	4. Lock side rails up on side of bed opposite from where clean linen is stacked.	
—	—	—	5. Raise bed to comfortable working position. Lower side rail on your side of bed.	
—	—	—	6. Loosen all top linen from foot of bed. Remove bedspread and blanket separately. Without shaking, fold each and place over back of chair if they are to be reused. If they are soiled, hold them away from your uniform and place in linen bag.	
—	—	—	7. Leave top sheet on client or cover client with a bath blanket, then remove and discard top sheet.	
—	—	—	8. Loosen bottom sheet on your side. Lower head of bed to flat position. If client cannot tolerate flat position, lower head of bed as far as client can tolerate.	
—	—	—	9. Help client roll onto side facing away from you. Have client grasp side rail to assist. Adjust pillow under head.	
—	—	—	10. Tightly fan-fold soiled draw sheet and tuck under buttocks, back, and shoulders. Repeat with soiled bottom sheet and tuck under client. Do not fan-fold mattress pad unless it is soiled.	
—	—	—	11. Place clean bottom sheet on bed. Unfold lengthwise so bottom edge is even with end of mattress and vertical center crease is at center of bed.	
—	—	—	12. Bring sheet's bottom edge over mattress sides and fanfold top of sheet toward center of mattress and place next to client.	
—	—	—	13. Tuck top edge of sheet under mattress. Miter the corner on your side (as in Procedure 32-8). Tuck remaining portion of sheet under mattress. Note: If contour sheets are used, fit elastic edges under corner of mattress.	

Excellent

Satisfactory

Needs Practice

PROCEDURE 32-9
MAKING AN OCCUPIED BED (Continued)

Comments

14. Place draw sheet on bed with the center fold at center of bed. Position sheet so it will extend from client's back to below the buttocks. Fan-fold the top edge and place next to client. Tuck excess under mattress.

15. Lock side rails up and move to opposite side of bed.

16. Lower side rail. Help client roll over folds of linen onto other side.

17. Move pillow under client's head.

18. Remove soiled linen by folding into a square or bundle, with soiled side turned in. Place in linen bag.

19. Grasp edge of fan-folded bottom sheet and pull from under client.

20. Tuck top of sheet under top of mattress. Miter top corner.

21. Facing bed, pull bottom sheet tight, and tuck excess linen under mattress from top to bottom.

22. Unfold draw sheet by grasping at center. Tuck excess tightly under mattress. Tuck the middle first, then top, and finally the bottom.

23. Help client to center of bed.

24. Raise side rail if necessary, and move to side of bed where remainder of linen is stored.

25. Place top sheet over client with center crease lengthwise at center of bed with seam side up. Unfold sheet from head to toe.

26. Have client grasp top edge of clean top sheet. Remove bath blanket or soiled top linen by pulling from beneath clean top sheet.

27. Discard in linen bag.

28. Complete top covers as described in Procedure 32-8.

29. Wash hands.

Name Fallan Pryor Date 8/31/05

Unit _____ Position _____

Instructor/Evaluator: _____ Position _____

Excellent	Satisfactory	Needs Practice	PROCEDURE 33-1 **USING BODY MECHANICS TO MOVE CLIENTS**	Comments
			Goal: To prevent injury to the nurse's musculoskeletal system and to prevent injury to clients during transfer.	

				Comments
—	⎮	—	1. Wash hands.	
—	⎮	—	2. Plan movement before doing it:	
—	⎮	—	a. Lock wheels on bed, stretcher, or wheelchair.	
—	⎮	—	b. Allow client to assist during move.	
—	⎮	—	c. Use mechanical aids (e.g., lifters, slide boards, body mobilizers) or additional personnel to move heavy clients.	8/31/05
			d. Slide, push, or pull client rather than lifting and carrying when possible.	Riley Ren
—	⎮	—	e. Tighten abdominal and gluteal muscles before lifting or moving client.	
—	⎮	—	f. Use smooth, rhythmic, coordinated movements.	
—	⎮	—	g. Plan movements before beginning when another person is assisting.	
—	⎮	—	3. Begin all movements with body aligned and balanced:	
—	⎮	—	a. Face client to be moved, and pivot your entire body without twisting your back.	
—	⎮	—	b. Place both feet flat on floor, knees slightly bent, with one foot slightly in front of the other or one step apart.	
—	⎮	—	c. Bend knees to lower center of gravity toward client to be moved.	
—	⎮	—	4. When possible, elevate adjustable beds to waist level, and lower side rails.	
—	⎮	—	5. Carry objects close to body, and stand as close as possible to work area.	

Name Fallan Pryor   Date 9/21/05

Unit _____   Position _____

Instructor/Evaluator: _____   Position _____

PROCEDURE 33-2
POSITIONING A CLIENT IN BED

Goal: To maintain proper body alignment for optimal ventilation and lung expansion and prevention of deformities of musculoskeletal system

Excellent	Satisfactory	Needs Practice		Comments

Moving a Client Up in Bed (One Nurse)

1. Identify client and any positioning restrictions. Explain procedure and rationale to client.
2. Lower head of bed to flat position, and raise level of bed to comfortable working height.
3. Remove all pillows from under client. Leave one at head of bed.
4. Instruct client to bend legs and put feet flat on bed.
5. Place your feet in broad stance with one foot in front of the other. Flex your knees and thighs.
6. Place one arm under client's shoulders and one arm under thighs. Keep head up and back straight.
7. Rock back and forth on front and back legs to count of three. On third count, have client push with feet as you lift and pull client up in bed.
8. Elevate head of bed and place pillows under head. Raise side rails and lower bed to lowest level.

Moving a Helpless Client Up in Bed (Two Nurses)

1. Identify client and any mobility restrictions. Explain procedure and rationale to client.
2. Lower head of bed to flat position, and raise level of bed to comfortable working height.
3. Remove all pillows from under client. Leave one at head of bed.
4. One nurse stands on each side of bed with legs positioned for wide base of support and one foot slightly in front of the other.
5. Each nurse rolls up and grasps edges of turn sheet close to client's shoulders and buttocks.
6. Flex knees and hips. Tighten abdominal and gluteal muscles, and keep back straight.

PROCEDURE 33-2
POSITIONING A CLIENT IN BED (Continued)

Excellent	Satisfactory	Needs Practice		Comments

7. Rock back and forth on front and back leg to count of three. On third count, both nurses shift weight to front leg as they simultaneously lift client toward head of bed.

8. Elevate head of bed and place pillows under client's head. Adjust other positioning pillows as necessary. Put up side rails, and lower bed to lowest level.

Positioning Client in Side-Lying Position

1. Identify client and note any mobility restrictions. Lower head of bed as flat as client can tolerate.

2. Elevate and lock side rail on side client will face when turned.

3. Using draw sheet, move client to edge of bed, opposite the side on which he or she will be turned.

4. Place arm that client will turn toward away from his or her body. Fold other arm across chest.

5. Flex client's knee that will not be next to mattress after turn. Have client reach toward side rail with opposite arm.

6. Assume a broad stance with knees slightly flexed.

7. Using a draw sheet, gently pull client over on side.

8. Align client properly, and place pillows behind back and under head.

9. Pull shoulder blade forward and out from under client. Support client's upper arm with pillow.

10. Place pillow lengthwise between client's legs from thighs to foot.

Logrolling

1. Obtain assistance of two or three other nurses.

2. All nurses stand on same side of bed, with feet apart, one foot slightly ahead of the other. Flex knees and hips.

3. Use one pillow to support client's head during and after turn.

4. Place pillows between client's legs.

5. Instruct client to fold arms over chest and keep body stiff.

6. Reach across client and support head, thorax, trunk, and legs. On count of three, roll client in one coordinated movement to lateral position.

POSITIONING A CLIENT IN BED (Continued)

Excellent	Satisfactory	Needs Practice		Comments
—	✓	—	7. Support client in alignment with pillows as described in Side-Lying Position. Clients with suspected or known cervical spinal injuries should wear cervical collar to prevent injury to the spinal cord whenever turning or moving in bed.	

Name Feilan Pryor   Date 9/21/05

Unit _____   Position _____

Instructor/Evaluator: _____ Position _____

PROCEDURE 33-3

PROVIDING RANGE OF MOTION EXERCISES

Goal: To maintain joint mobility, improve or maintain muscle strength, and prevent muscle atrophy and contractures.

Excellent	Satisfactory	Needs Practice		Comments
			1. Identify client and client's movement limitations. Explain procedure and purpose to client.	
			2. Position client on back with head of bed as flat as possible. Elevate bed to comfortable working height.	
			3. Stand on side of bed of joints to be exercised. Uncover limb to be exercised only.	
			4. Perform exercises slowly and gently, providing support by holding areas proximal and distal to the joint.	
			5. Repeat each exercise five times. Discontinue or decrease ROM if client complains of discomfort or muscle spasm.	
			6. Neck:	
			a. Move chin to chest.	
			b. Bend head toward back.	
			c. Tilt head toward each shoulder.	
			d. Rotate head in circular motion.	
			e. Return head to erect position.	
			7. Shoulder:	
			a. Raise client's arm from side to above head.	
			b. Abduct and rotate shoulder by raising arm above head with palm up.	
			c. Adduct shoulder by moving arm across body as far as possible.	
			d. Rotate shoulder internally and externally by flexing elbow and moving forearm so that palm touches mattress; then reverse the motion so that back of client's hand touches mattress.	
			e. Move shoulder in a full circle.	
			8. Elbow:	
			a. Bend elbow so that forearm moves toward shoulder.	
			b. Hyperextend elbow as far as possible.	
			9. Wrist and hand:	

PROCEDURE 33-3
PROVIDING RANGE OF MOTION EXERCISES (Continued)

Excellent	Satisfactory	Needs Practice		Comments

a. Move hand toward inner aspect of forearm.

b. Bend dorsal surface of hand backward.

c. Abduct wrist by bending toward thumb.

d. Adduct wrist by bending toward fifth finger.

e. Make a fist, then extend the fingers.

f. Spread fingers apart, then together.

g. Move thumb across hand to base of fifth finger.

10. Hip and knee:

    a. Lift leg and bend knee toward chest.

    b. Abduct and adduct leg, moving leg laterally away from body and returning to medial position.

    c. Internally and externally rotate hip by turning leg inward, then outward.

    d. Take special care to support joints of larger limbs.

11. Ankle and foot:

    a. Dorsiflex foot by moving foot so toes point upward.

    b. Plantar flex by moving foot so toes point downward.

    c. Curl toes down, then extend.

    d. Spread toes apart, then bring together.

    e. Invert by turning sole of foot medially.

    f. Evert by turning sole of foot laterally.

12. Move to other side of bed and repeat exercises.

13. Reposition client to position of comfort.

14. Document ROM.

Name Fallan Pryor   Date 9/21/05

Unit ___   Position ___

Instructor/Evaluator: ___   Position ___

PROCEDURE 33-4
ASSISTING WITH AMBULATION

Goal: To promote safe ambulation free of falls or injury.

Comments

Excellent	Satisfactory	Needs Practice		
			1. Identify client. Explain procedure and purpose of ambulation to client. Decide together how far and where to walk.	
			2. Place bed in lowest position.	
			3. Assist client to sitting position on side of bed. Assess for dizziness or faintness. Obtain orthostatic vital signs if complaints are present. Allow client to remain in this position until he or she feels secure.	
			4. Help client with clothing and footwear.	

One Nurse

1. Wrap transfer belt around client's waist (optional according to assessment).
2. Assist client to standing position, and assess client's balance. Return to bed or transfer to chair if very weak or unsteady. Be sure client does not grasp your neck for support, but places his or her hands around your shoulders or at your waist.
3. Position yourself behind client while supporting him or her by waist or transfer belt.
4. Take several steps forward with client, assessing strength and balance. Encourage client to use good posture and to look ahead, not down at feet.
5. Ambulate for planned distance or time. If client becomes weak or dizzy, return to bed or assist to chair.
6. If client begins to fall, place your feet wide apart with one foot in front. Support client by pulling his or her weight backward against your body. Lower gently to floor, protecting head.

Two Nurses

1. Assist client to sitting position as described.
2. Assist client to standing position with one nurse on each side.

PROCEDURE 33-4
ASSISTING WITH AMBULATION (Continued)

Excellent	Satisfactory	Needs Practice		Comments
			3. One nurse grasps the transfer belt to support the client. The other nurse may carry and manage equipment.	
			4. Walk with client using slow, even steps. Assess strength and balance. Encourage client to look forward rather than down at floor.	
			Using a Walker	
			1. Assist client to standing position. One hand remains on the arm of the chair or bed as client assumes an upright posture.	
			2. Have client grasp walker handles. Client moves walker ahead 6 to 8 inches placing all four feet of walker on floor. Client moves forward to walker.	
			3. Nurse should walk close behind and slightly to side of client.	
			4. Repeat above sequence until walk is complete.	

Name Fallan Pryor   Date 9/21/05

Unit _____   Position _____

Instructor/Evaluator: _____   Position _____

Excellent	Satisfactory	Needs Practice		Comments

PROCEDURE 33-5
HELPING CLIENTS WITH CRUTCHWALKING

Goal: To increase client's level of activity safely after musculoskeletal injury.

Four-Point Gait

____	____	____	1. Instruct client to stand erect, facing forward in tripod position. Client places crutch tips 6 inches in front of feet and 6 inches to side of each foot.
____	____	____	2. Client moves right crutch forward 6 inches.
____	____	____	3. Client moves left foot forward to level of right crutch.
____	____	____	4. Client moves left crutch forward 4 to 6 inches.
____	____	____	5. Client moves right foot forward to level of left crutch.
____	____	____	6. Repeat sequence.

Three-Point Gait

____	____	____	1. Beginning in tripod position, client moves both crutches and affected leg forward.
____	____	____	2. Client moves stronger leg forward.
____	____	____	3. Repeat sequence. Client must bear entire weight on stronger leg to perform this gait.

Two-Point gait

____	____	____	1. Beginning in the tripod position, client moves left crutch and right foot forward.
____	____	____	2. Client moves right crutch and left foot forward.
____	____	____	3. Repeat sequence.

Swing-To Gait

____	____	____	1. Client forms tripod position and moves both crutches forward.
____	____	____	2. Client lifts legs and swings to crutches, supporting body weight on crutches.

Swing Through Gait

____	____	____	1. Client forms tripod position and moves both crutches forward.

HELPING CLIENTS WITH CRUTCHWALKING (Continued)

Excellent	Satisfactory	Needs Practice		Comments

Excellent   **Satisfactory**   **Needs Practice**   **Comments**

2. Client lifts legs and swings through and ahead of crutches, supporting weight on crutches.

Climbing Stairs

1. Use one crutch and the railing. Beginning in tripod position facing stairs, client transfers body weight to crutches and holds onto the railing.
2. Client places unaffected leg on stair.
3. Client transfers body weight to unaffected leg.
4. Client moves crutches and affected leg to stair.
5. Repeat sequence to top of stairs.

74

Name Feulen Pryor   Date 9/21/05

Unit _____   Position _____

Instructor/Evaluator: _____   Position _____

CHECKLIST 33-6
TRANSFERRING A CLIENT TO A STRETCHER

Excellent	Satisfactory	Needs Practice	**Goal:** To transfer client without injury to client or nurse.	Comments
—	|	—	1. Identify client. Explain procedure and purpose to client.	
—	|	—	2. Place stretcher parallel to bed. Raise bed to same level as stretcher. Lower side rails. Lock wheels on bed.	
—	|	—	3. One or two nurses stand on side of bed without stretcher. Two nurses stand on side of bed with stretcher.	
—	|	—	4. Loosen draw sheet on both sides of bed.	
—	|	—	5. Nurses on side without stretcher help client to move toward them onto his or her side, using draw sheet to pull client closer to stretcher.	
—	↓	—	6. Nurses on stretcher side of bed slide transfer board under draw sheet and under client's buttocks and back.	
—	|	—	7. Slide client onto transfer board into supine position. Place client's arms across chest.	
—	↓	—	8. Wrap end of draw sheet over curved end of transfer board, and slide client onto stretcher on count of three.	
—	|	—	9. Roll client slightly up onto side, and pull transfer board out from under him or her.	
—	↓	—	10. Lock side rails up on bed side of stretcher, and move stretcher away from bed.	
—	|	—	11. Place sheet over client, and lock safety belts across client's chest and waist. Adjust head of stretcher according to client limitations.	

Name Fallan Pryor   Date 9/21/05

Unit _____   Position _____

Instructor/Evaluator: _____   Position _____

Excellent	Satisfactory	Needs Practice	PROCEDURE 33-7 **TRANSFERRING A CLIENT TO A WHEELCHAIR**	Comments
			Goal: To increase mobility and independence by using wheelchair.	
—		—	1. Identify client and explain procedure.	
—		—	2. Position wheelchair at 45-degree angle or parallel to bed. Remove footrests and lock brakes.	
—		—	3. Lock bed brakes, lower bed to lowest level, and raise head of bed as far as client can tolerate.	
—		—	4. Assist client to side-lying position, facing the side of bed on which he or she will sit. Lower side rail, and stand near client's hips with foot near head of bed in front of and apart from other foot.	
—		—	5. Apply transfer belt. Grip belt to assist with transfer.	
—		—	6. Swing client's legs over side of bed. At the same time, pivot on your back leg to lift client's trunk and shoulders. Keep back straight, and avoid twisting.	
—		—	7. Stand in front of client, and assess for balance and dizziness.	
—		—	8. Help client to don robe and nonskid footwear.	
—		—	9. Spread your feet apart, and flex your hips and knees.	
—		—	10. Have client slide buttocks to edge of bed until feet touch floor.	
—		—	11. Rock back and forth until client stands on a count of three.	
—		—	12. Brace your front knee against client's weak knee as client stands.	
—		—	13. Pivot on back foot until client feels wheelchair against back of legs, keeping your knee against the client's knee.	
—		—	14. Instruct client to place hands on chair armrests for support. Flex your knees and hips as you assist client into chair.	
—	✓	—	15. Adjust foot pedal and leg supports.	
—	—	—	16. Assess client's alignment in chair. Provide call light.	

Name _Fallon Pryor_   Date _9/21/05_

Unit _____   Position _____

Instructor/Evaluator: _N Anderson RN MSN_   Position _____

Excellent	Satisfactory	Needs Practice	PROCEDURE 33-8 **TRANSFERING CLIENT FROM BED TO CHAIR USING HYDRAULIC LIFT**	Comments
			Goal: To transfer a client safely from a bed to a chair using a hydraulic lift, without which a safe transfer would not be possible.	
—	—	—	1. Identify client and any mobility restrictions. Explain procedure and purpose to client.	
—	—	—	2. Place fabric sling evenly under client.	
—	—	—	3. Position hydraulic lift so the frame can be centered over the client. Attach the fabric sling to the frame. Note manufacturer's instructions for specifics of how sling should be attached to the frame.	
—	—	—	4. Have a nurse on each side of the hydraulic lift. Warn the client that he or she will be lifted from the bed. Support head and heavy casts as needed. Engage the hydraulic system to raise client from bed.	
—	—	—	5. Carefully wheel client in hydraulic lift away from the bed, supporting limbs as needed. Position over chair, and gently lower to chair using the hydraulic mechanism.	
—	—	—	6. The sling remains in place under the client and is reattached to the frame when the client is moved back to bed.	

Name Fallon Pryor

Date 11/2/08

Unit

Position

Instructor/Evaluator: Of Hey Rn

Position

Excellent	Satisfactory	Needs Practice	PROCEDURE 34-1 **MONITORING WITH PULSE OXIMETRY**	Comments

Goal: To monitor arterial oxygen saturation (SaO_2) noninvasively and to detect promptly deviations from normal.

Excellent	Satisfactory	Needs Practice		Comments
✓	—	—	1. Select appropriate type of sensor, considering client's weight, level of activity, whether infection control is a concern, allergies, and the anticipated duration of monitoring.	
	—	—	2. Explain purpose of procedure to client and family.	
	—	—	3. Instruct client to breathe normally.	
	—	—	4. Select appropriate site to place sensor. Avoid using lower extremities that may have compromised circulation or extremities receiving infusions or other invasive monitoring. Consider use of nasal sensor or forehead sensor for clients with poor tissue perfusion.	
	—	—	5. Remove nail polish or acrylic nail from digit to be used.	
	—	—	6. Attach sensor probe, and connect it to the pulse oximeter. Make sure the photosensors are accurately aligned.	
	—	—	7. Watch for pulse-sensing bar on face of oximeter to fluctuate with each pulsation and reflect pulse strength. Double-check machine pulsations with client's radial or apical pulse.	
	—	—	8. If continuous pulse oximetry is desired, set alarm limits on monitor to reflect high and low oxygen saturation and pulse rates. Ensure that the alarms are audible before leaving client. Inspect sensor site every 4 hours for tissue irritation or pressure.	
	—	—	9. Read saturation on monitor, and document as appropriate with all relevant information on client's chart. Report SaO_2 less than 93% to physician.	

Name Fallan Pryor

Date _____

Unit _____

Position _____

Instructor/Evaluator: Gurney RN on

Position _____

Excellent	Satisfactory	Needs Practice	PROCEDURE 34-2 **TEACHING COUGHING AND DEEP BREATHING EXERCISES**	Comments
			Goal: To facilitate respiratory functioning by increasing expansion, preventing alveolar collapse, and promoting expectoration of secretions.	
	1/05		**Deep Breathing** 1. Assist client to Fowler's or sitting position.	
__	__	__	2. Have client place hands palm down, with middle fingers touching, along lower border of rib cage.	
__	__	__	3. Ask client to inhale slowly through the nose, feeling middle fingers separate. Hold breath for 2 or 3 seconds.	
__	__	__	4. Have client exhale slowly through mouth. Repeat three to five times.	
__	__	__	**Controlled Coughing** 1. If adventitious breath sounds or sputum is present, have client take a deep breath, hold for 3 seconds, and cough deeply two or three times. Stand to client's side to ensure the cough is not directed at you. Client must cough deeply, not just clear the throat.	
__	__	__	2. If client has an abdominal or chest incision that will cause pain during coughing, instruct client to hold a pillow firmly over the incision (splinting) when coughing.	
__	__	__	3. Instruct, reinforce, and supervise deep-breathing and coughing exercises every 2 to 3 hours postoperatively.	
__	__	__	4. Document procedure.	

Name Fallon Pryor

Date _____

Unit _____

Position _____

Instructor/Evaluator: G Turner RN

Position _____

PROCEDURE 34-3

PROMOTING BREATHING WITH THE INCENTIVE SPIROMETER

Goal: To improve pulmonary ventilation and oxygenation and to loosen respiratory secretions.

Excellent	Satisfactory	Needs Practice		Comments
	1/08		1. Verify the physician's order, and identify the client.	
			2. Wash hands.	
			3. Assist client to high Fowler's or sitting position.	
			4. Determine the volume to set incentive spirometry goal based on calculated lung volumes. Use chart or have respiratory therapy calculate. Set volume indicator.	
			5. Instruct client in procedure:	
			a. Seal lips tightly around mouthpiece.	
			b. Inhale slowly and deeply through mouth. Hold breath for 2 or 3 seconds.	
			c. Have client observe his or her progress by watching the balls elevate or lights go on, depending on type of equipment used.	
			d. Exhale slowly around mouthpiece and breathe normally for several breaths.	
			6. Repeat procedure 5 to 10 times every 1 to 2 hours per physician's orders.	

Name _____   Date _____

Unit _____   Position _____

Instructor/Evaluator: _____   Position _____

PROCEDURE 34-4
MONITORING PEAK FLOW

Goal: To measure peak expiratory flow rate (PEFR) to assess respiratory function.

Columns: Excellent | Satisfactory | Needs Practice

Comments

1. Verify physician's order, and identify the client.
2. Explain the purpose of peak flow monitoring to client and family.
3. Place indicator at base of numbered scale. Have client stand up.
4. Tell client to take deep breath. Place meter in his or her mouth. Client should close lips around the mouthpiece. Remind client to keep tongue out of the hole.
5. Tell client to exhale as fast and as hard as he or she can, keeping a tight fit around the mouthpiece.
6. Repeat Steps 2 through 4 twice more, and record the highest peak flow obtained in the three attempts.
7. To determine "personal best" when beginning peak flow monitoring, obtain peak flow measurements in the morning and again in the evening over a 2-week period of good asthma control. Client should take measurements before using bronchodilators.
8. Healthcare provider will calculate zones based on percentage of personal best (green 80%-100%; yellow 50%-80%; red below 50%) and give instruction for what to do in each zone.
9. Encourage client to comply with twice-a-day (morning and evening) monitoring before bronchodilator therapy and to follow healthcare provider's instructions for peak flows in each zone. Follow Steps 2 through 5.

Name Fallan Pryon   Date 11/2/05

Unit _____   Position _____

Instructor/Evaluator: _____   Position _____

PROCEDURE 34-5

ADMINISTERING OXYGEN BY NASAL CANNULA OR MASK

Goal: To deliver low to moderate levels of oxygen to relieve hypoxia.

Excellent	Satisfactory	Needs Practice		Comments
			1. Review chart for physician's order for oxygen to include method of delivery, flow rate, duration of therapy, and client identification.	
			2. Wash hands.	
			3. Explain procedure to client. Explain that oxygen will ease dyspnea or discomfort, and inform client concerning safety precautions associated with oxygen use. If client is using the cannula, encourage him or her to breathe through the nose.	
			4. Assist client to semi or high Fowler's position if tolerated.	
			5. Insert flowmeter into wall outlet. Attach oxygen tubing to nozzle on flowmeter; if using a high O_2 flow, attach humidifier.	
			6. Turn on the oxygen at the prescribed rate. Check that oxygen is flowing through tubing.	
			7. Cannula:	
			a. Place cannula prongs into nares.	
			b. Wrap tubing over and behind ears.	
			c. Adjust plastic slide under chin until cannula fits snugly.	
			8. Mask:	
			a. Place mask on face, applying from nose and over chin.	
			b. Adjust the metal rim over the nose, and contour the mask to the face.	
			c. Adjust elastic band around head so mask fits snugly.	
			9. Assess for proper functioning of equipment, and observe client's initial response to therapy.	
			10. Monitor continuous therapy by assessing for pressure areas on the skin and nares every 2 hours and rechecking flow rate every 4 to 8 hours.	
			11. Document procedure and observations.	

82

Excellent	Satisfactory	Needs Practice	PROCEDURE 34-6 **MONITORING A CLIENT WITH A CHEST DRAINAGE SYSTEM**	Comments
			Goal: To monitor respiratory status of client with a chest tube and to ensure that the drainage system is functioning adequately.	
___	___	___	1. Confirm physician's order, including amount of suction.	
___	___	___	2. Assist client to semi or high Fowler's position.	
___	___	___	3. Assess insertion site of chest tube. Note and document amount and color of drainage on dressing around insertion site. Feel insertion site for crepitus. Document any crepitus found. Reinforce insertion dressing as needed.	
___	___	___	4. Assess status of chest tubing. Be sure tubing remains at level of client and no dependent loops are present. Assess that there are no visible clots in tubing. You may gently "milk" the clots to encourage movement into the drainage system, but never strip chest tubing.	
___	___	___	5. Assess drainage collection chamber. Be sure to keep chest drainage system upright. Assess for amount, color, and character of drainage. Mark collection chamber to reflect accurately amount of drainage accumulated during your shift.	
___	___	___	6. Assess suction chamber. Make sure the water level in suction chamber is at the prescribed amount of suction and that it is connected to the wall suction, which is turned on to continuous suction.	
___	___	___	7. Assess system for air leaks. Check all external connections (i.e., chest tube connection to drainage system, suction tubing connection to drainage system). Examine water seal chamber as client breathes normally and as client coughs.	
___	___	___	8. Encourage client to cough, deep breathe, and use an incentive spirometer frequently. Provide analgesics as necessary.	
___	___	___	9. If chest tube becomes expelled, do not leave client. Cover opening where chest tube was inserted with sterile 4x4 gauze, and keep direct pressure on the site. Send a colleague to call the physician immediately.	
___	___	___	10. Document chest tube drainage, patency of chest tubes, the presence of an air leak, the amount of suction, pain level, status of the dressing, and respiratory status.	

Name _____ Date _____

Unit _____ Position _____

Instructor/Evaluator: _____ Position _____

Excellent	Satisfactory	Needs Practice	PROCEDURE 34-7 **PROVIDING TRACHEOSTOMY CARE**	
			Goal: To maintain airway patency by removing mucus and encrusted secretions and to prevent infection or skin breakdown at stoma site.	**Comments**
——	——	——	1. Validate physician's order, and identify client.	
——	——	——	2. Wash hands and don gloves.	
——	——	——	3. Explain procedure to client. Place client in semi to high Fowler's position.	
——	——	——	4. Suction tracheostomy tube. Before discarding gloves, remove soiled tracheostomy dressing, and discard with catheter inside glove. *Note: Follow Procedure 34-8, but insert catheter through tracheostomy tube and advance about 10 to 12 cm in an adult.*	
——	——	——	5. Replace oxygen or humidification source, and encourage client to deep breathe as you prepare sterile supplies.	
——	——	——	6. Open sterile tracheostomy kit. Don sterile gloves. Pour normal saline into one basin and hydrogen peroxide into the second. Open several sterile cotton-tipped applicators and one sterile precut tracheostomy dressing, and place on sterile field. If kit does not contain tracheostomy ties, cut two 15-inch pieces of twill tape and set aside.	
——	——	——	7. Remove oxygen or humidity source. Note: For tracheostomy tube with inner cannula, complete Steps 8 to 25. For tracheostomy tube without inner cannula or plugged with a button, complete Steps 14 to 25.	
——	——	——	8. Unplug inner cannula by turning counterclockwise. Remove inner cannula.	
——	——	——	9. Place inner cannula in basin with hydrogen peroxide.	
——	——	——	10. Replace oxygen source over or near outer cannula.	
——	——	——	11. Clean lumen and sides of inner cannula using pipe cleaners or sterile brush.	
——	——	——	12. Rinse inner cannula thoroughly by agitating in normal saline for several seconds.	
——	——	——	13. Remove oxygen source and replace inner cannula into outer cannula. "Lock" by turning clockwise until the two blue dots align. Replace oxygen or humidity source.	

Excellent	Satisfactory	Needs Practice		Comments

——	——	——	14. Clean stoma under faceplate with circular motion using hydrogen peroxide-soaked cotton applicators. Clean dried secretions from all exposed outer cannula surfaces.	
——	——	——	15. Remove foaming secretions using normal saline-soaked cotton-tipped applicators.	
——	——	——	16. Pat moist surfaces dry with 4x4-inch gauze.	
——	——	——	17. Place dry, sterile, precut tracheostomy dressing around tracheostomy stoma and under faceplate. Do not use cut 4x4-inch gauze.	
——	——	——	18. If tracheostomy ties are to be changed, have an assistant don a sterile glove and hold the tracheostomy tube in place.	
——	——	——	19. Cut a 1/2-inch slit approximately 1 inch from one end of both clean tracheostomy ties. Fold back on itself 1 inch of the tie, and cut a small slit in the middle.	
——	——	——	20. Remove and discard soiled tracheostomy ties.	
——	——	——	21. Thread end of tie through cut slit in tie. Pull tight.	
——	——	——	22. Repeat Step 21 with second tie.	
——	——	——	23. Bring both ties together at one side of client's neck. Assess that ties are only tight enough to allow one finger between tie and neck. Use two square knots to secure the ties. Trim excess tie length.	
——	——	——	24. Remove gloves and discard disposable equipment. Label with date and time, and store reusable supplies.	
——	——	——	25. Assist client to comfortable position and offer oral hygiene.	
——	——	——	26. Wash hands and document the procedure and observations.	

Name _____   Date _____

Unit _____   Position _____

Instructor/Evaluator: _____   Position _____

Excellent	Satisfactory	Needs Practice	PROCEDURE 34-8 **SUCTIONING SECRETIONS FROM AIRWAYS**	
			Goal: To maintain patent airway by removing excess secretions.	**Comments**
___	___	___	1. Verify physician's order, and identify client.	
___	___	___	2. Wash hands.	
___	___	___	3. Explain procedure and purpose to client.	
___	___	___	4. Position the client.	
___	___	___	a. Position conscious client with an intact gag reflex in semi Fowler's position.	
___	___	___	b. Position the unconscious client in a side-lying position facing you.	
___	___	___	5. Turn suction device on and adjust pressure: infants and children, 50 to 75 mm Hg; adults, 100 to 120 mm Hg.	
___	___	___	6. Open and prepare sterile suction catheter kit.	
___	___	___	a. Unfold sterile cup, touching only the outside. Place on bedside table.	
___	___	___	b. Pour sterile saline into cup.	
___	___	___	7. Preoxygenate client with 100% oxygen. Hyperinflate with manual resuscitation bag.	
___	___	___	8. Don sterile gloves. If kit provides only one glove, place on dominant hand. You may use a clean disposable glove on the nondominant hand to protect yourself from exposure to mucous membranes and sputum.	
___	___	___	9. Pick up catheter with dominant hand. Pick up connecting tubing with nondominant hand. Attach catheter to tubing without contaminating sterile hand.	
___	___	___	10. Place catheter end into cup of saline. Test functioning of equipment by applying thumb from nondominant hand over open port to create suction. Return catheter to sterile field.	
___	___	___	11. Insert catheter into trachea through nostril, nasal trumpet, or artificial airway during inspiration.	
___	___	___	12. Advance catheter until you feel resistance. Retract catheter 1 cm before applying suction. Note: Client usually will cough when catheter enters trachea.	

SUCTIONING SECRETIONS FROM AIRWAYS (Continued)

Excellent	Satisfactory	Needs Practice		Comments
___	___	___	13. Apply suction by placing thumb of nondominant hand over open port. Rotate the catheter with your dominant hand as you withdraw the catheter. This should take 5 to 10 seconds.	
___	___	___	14. Hyperoxygenate and hyperinflate using manual resuscitation bag for a full minute between subsequent suction passes.	
___	___	___	15. Rinse catheter thoroughly with saline.	
___	___	___	16. Repeat Steps 11 to 15 until airway is clear.	
___	___	___	17. Without applying suction, insert the catheter gently along one side of the mouth. Advance to the oropharynx.	
___	___	___	18. Apply suction for 5 to 10 seconds as you rotate and withdraw catheter.	
___	___	___	19. Allow 1 to 2 minutes between passes for the client to ventilate.	
___	___	___	20. Repeat Steps 17 and 18 as necessary to clear oropharynx.	
___	___	___	21. Rinse catheter and tubing by suctioning saline through.	
___	___	___	22. Remove gloves by holding catheter with dominant hand and pulling glove off inside-out. Catheter will remain coiled inside glove. Pull other glove off inside-out. Dispose of in trash receptacle.	
___	___	___	23. Turn off suction device.	
___	___	___	24. Assist client to comfortable position. Offer assistance with oral and nasal hygiene. Replace oxygen device if used.	
___	___	___	25. Dispose of disposable supplies.	
___	___	___	26. Wash hands	
___	___	___	27. Ensure that sterile suction kit is available at head of bed.	
___	___	___	28. Document procedure and observations.	

Name _____ Date _____

Unit _____ Position _____

Instructor/Evaluator: _____ Position _____

Excellent	Satisfactory	Needs Practice	PROCEDURE 34-9 **MANAGING AN OBSTRUCTED AIRWAY** **(HEIMLICH MANEUVER)**	Comments
			Goal: To remove a foreign body from obstructing the airway to prevent anoxia and cardiopulmonary arrest.	
			Conscious Child or Adult	
___	___	___	1. Client is standing or sitting.	
___	___	___	2. Stand behind client.	
___	___	___	3. Wrap your arms around client's waist.	
___	___	___	4. Make a fist with one hand. Place thumb side of fist against client's abdomen, above the navel but below the xiphoid process.	
___	___	___	5. Grasp fist with other hand.	
___	___	___	6. Press fist into abdomen with a quick upward thrust.	
___	___	___	7. Repeat distinct separate thrust until the client expels the foreign body or becomes unconscious.	
			Unconscious Client (Heimlich Maneuver, Abdominal Thrust)	
___	___	___	1. Client is lying on ground.	
___	___	___	2. Turn client on back and call for help. Activate emergency response system (911).	
___	___	___	3. If there is no effective breathing, attempt to provide two rescue breaths. If unsuccessful, reposition head and try to ventilate again.	
			4. Finger sweep:	
___	___	___	a. Use tongue-jaw lift to open mouth.	
___	___	___	b. Insert index finger inside cheek and sweep to base of tongue. Use hooking motion if possible to dislodge and remove the foreign body. Avoid finger sweeps in infants and children because you can easily push the foreign body further into the airway. Remove only if clearly visible and easy to reach.	
___	___	___	5. Straddle client's thighs or kneel to the side of thighs.	
___	___	___	6. Place heel of one hand on epigastric area, midline above the navel but below the xiphoid process.	
___	___	___	7. Place second hand on top of first hand.	

PROCEDURE 34-9
MANAGING AN OBSTRUCTED AIRWAY
(Continued)

Excellent	Satisfactory	Needs Practice		Comments

——— ——— ——— 8. Press heel of hand into abdomen with a quick upward thrust.

——— ——— ——— 9. Repeat abdominal thrusts five times.

——— ——— ——— 10. If airway is still obstructed, attempt to ventilate using mouth-to-mouth respiration and head tilt/chin lift.

——— ——— ——— 11. Repeat Steps 6 through 9 until successful.

**Children Younger than One Year of Age
(Back Blows and Chest Thrusts)**

——— ——— ——— 1. Straddle infant over your arm with head lower than trunk.

——— ——— ——— 2. Support head by holding jaw firmly in your hand.

——— ——— ——— 3. Rest your forearm on your thigh and deliver five back blows with the heel of your hand between the infant's scapula.

——— ——— ——— 4. Place free hand on infant's back and support neck while turning to supine position.

——— ——— ——— 5. Place two fingers over sternum in same location as for external chest compression (one finger-width below nipple line).

——— ——— ——— 6. Administer five chest thrusts.

——— ——— ——— 7. Repeat Steps 1 through 6 until airway is not obstructed.

Children Older than 1 Year of Age

——— ——— ——— 1. Perform Heimlich maneuver with child standing, sitting, or lying as for adult but more gently.

——— ——— ——— 2. You may need to kneel behind child or have child stand on a table.

——— ——— ——— 3. Prevent foreign body airway obstruction in infants and children by teaching parents or caregivers to:

——— ——— ———   a. Restrict children from walking, running, or playing with food or foreign objects in their mouths.

——— ——— ———   b. Keep small objects (e.g., marbles, beads, beans) away from children younger than 3 years.

——— ——— ———   c. Avoid feeding popcorn and peanuts to children younger than 3 years, and cut other foods into small pieces.

——— ——— ——— 4. Instruct parents and caregivers in the management of foreign body airway obstruction.

PROCEDURE 34-9
MANAGING AN OBSTRUCTED AIRWAY
(Continued)

Excellent	Satisfactory	Needs Practice		Comments

Pregnant Women or Very Obese Adults (Chest Thrusts)

1. Stand behind client.
2. Bring your arms under client's armpits and around chest.
3. Make a fist and place thumb side against middle of sternum.
4. Grasp fist with other hand and deliver quick, backward thrust.
5. Repeat thrusts until airway is cleared.
6. Chest thrusts may be performed with client supine and hands positioned with heel over lower half of sternum. Administer separate, downward thrusts until airway is clear.

Name _____ Date _____

Unit _____ Position _____

Instructor/Evaluator: _____ Position _____

PROCEDURE 35-1
APPLYING ANTIEMBOLIC STOCKINGS

Goal: To supplement the action of muscle contraction and aid venous return from lower extremities.

Excellent	Satisfactory	Needs Practice		Comments

1. Position client in supine position for one half hour before applying stockings.
2. Provide for the client's privacy, and explain purpose of antiembolic stockings.
3. Measure for proper fit before first application. Measure length (heel to groin) and width (calf and thigh) and compare to manufacturer's printed material to ensure proper fit.
4. Make sure legs are dry or apply a light dusting of powder. Turn stocking inside out, tucking the foot inside.
5. Ease foot section over client's toe and heel, adjusting as necessary for proper fit.
6. Gently pull stocking over leg, removing all wrinkles
7. Assess toes for circulation and warmth. Check area at top of stocking for binding.
8. Antiembolic stockings should be removed at least twice daily.

Name _____ Date _____

Unit _____ Position _____

Instructor/Evaluator: _____ Position _____

Excellent	Satisfactory	Needs Practice	PROCEDURE 35-2 **APPLYING A SEQUENTIAL COMPRESSION DEVICE (SCD)**	Comments
			Goal: To promote venous return from legs to decrease the risk of deep vein thrombosis and pulmonary embolism.	
___	___	___	1. Identify client. Explain procedure and purpose to client.	
___	___	___	2. Provide for client's privacy.	
___	___	___	3. Measure leg to ensure proper sleeve sizing.	
___	___	___	a. Knee length: One size fits all.	
___	___	___	b. Thigh length: Measure length of leg from ankle to popliteal fossa. Measure circumference of thigh at the gluteal fold.	
___	___	___	4. Apply antiembolism stockings. Ensure that there are no wrinkles or folds (see Procedure 35-1). Use stockinette or ace wraps if unable to fit client with antiembolism stockings.	
___	___	___	5. Place client in supine position.	
___	___	___	6. Place a plastic sleeve under each leg so the opening is at the knee. If only one sleeve is required, leave the other sleeve in package, and connect to control unit.	
___	___	___	7. Fold outer section of the sleeve over the inner portion, and secure with Velcro tabs. Check sleeve fit. Two fingers should fit between the sleeve and leg.	
___	___	___	8. Connect tubing to control unit. The premarked arrows on the tubing from the sleeve and from the controller must be aligned to make adequate connection. Turn machine on.	
___	___	___	9. Adjust the control unit settings as necessary. Unit control is preset with sleeve cooling in "off" position and audible alarm in "on" position. Sleeve cooling should be in "on" position at all times except during surgery to preserve warmth for client. Ankle pressure should be set at 35 to 55 mm Hg.	
___	___	___	10. Recheck control unit settings whenever unit has been turned off.	
___	___	___	11. Respond to and promptly correct all "fault" indicator alarms. The control unit will sense four pressure "fault" conditions:	

PROCEDURE 35-2
APPLYING A SEQUENTIAL COMPRESSION DEVICE (SCD)
(Continued)

Excellent	Satisfactory	Needs Practice		Comments
___	___	___	a. Pressure failed to drop to zero during the cycle.	
___	___	___	b. Ankle pressure failed to reach 20 mm Hg.	
___	___	___	c. Ankle pressure exceeded 90 mm Hg.	
___	___	___	d. Internal diagnostics error has occurred.	
___	___	___	12. Document time and date of application. If SCD is applied to only one leg, document reason.	
___	___	___	13. Assess and document skin integrity every 8 hours.	
___	___	___	14. Remove sleeves and notify physician if client experiences tingling, numbness, or leg pain.	

Name _____   Date _____

Unit _____   Position _____

Instructor/Evaluator: _____   Position _____

Excellent	Satisfactory	Needs Practice	PROCEDURE 35-3 **ADMINISTERING CARDIOPULMONARY RESUSCITATION**	
			Goal: To restore cardiopulmonary functioning.	**Comments**
			One Rescuer—Adult Client	
___	___	___	1. Ask "Are your okay?" Assess to determine responsiveness. Shake gently.	
___	___	___	2. Call for help, or activate emergency response system (911).	
___	___	___	3. Turn client onto back while supporting head and neck. Place a cardiac board under the back, or place client on the floor.	
___	___	___	4. Open the airway:	
___	___	___	a. Use the head tilt/chin lift maneuver.	
___	___	___	b. Use the modified jaw thrust if a neck injury is suspected.	
___	___	___	5. Place your ear over client's mouth, and observe the chest for rising with respiration. *Listen, look, and feel* for breathing for 3 to 5 seconds.	
___	___	___	6. Pinch the client's nostrils with thumb and index finger of hand holding the forehead.	
___	___	___	7. Take a deep breath, and place your mouth around the client's mouth with a tight seal. If client wears dentures, they should remain in place.	
___	___	___	8. Ventilate two slow breaths. Each breath should take 2 seconds to deliver. Pause between breaths to allow for lung deflation and to take another deep breath.	
___	___	___	9. If client is breathing but still unresponsive, turn on to side (recovery position).	
___	___	___	10. Assess for carotid pulse for 5 to 10 seconds on the side next to which you are kneeling. Maintain head tilt with the other hand.	
___	___	___	11. If client is pulseless, start chest compressions.	
___	___	___	12. With the hand nearest client's legs, place middle and index fingers on lower ridge or near ribs, and move fingers up along ribs to the costalsternal notch (in center of lower chest).	

PROCEDURE 35-3

ADMINISTERING CARDIOPULMONARY RESUSCITATION
(Continued)

Excellent	Satisfactory	Needs Practice		Comments

13. Place middle finger on this notch and the index finger next to the middle finger on the lower end of the notch.

14. Place heel of other hand along the lower half of the sternum, next to the index finger.

15. Remove first hand from the notch and place heel of that hand parallel over the hand on the chest. Interlock fingers, keeping them off client's chest.

16. Keeping your hands on sternum, extend your arms, locking the elbows, with your shoulders directly over the client's chest.

17. Press down on the chest, depressing sternum 1.5 to 2 inches.

18. Completely release compression while maintaining your hand position. Repeat in a smooth rhythm 100 times/min.

19. Ventilate with 2 full breaths after every 15 chest compressions.

20. Repeat 4 cycles of 15 chest compressions and 2 ventilations.

21. Reassess for carotid pulse. If client is pulseless, continue CPR. Reassess for carotid pulse every few minutes without interrupting CPR for more than 7 seconds.

Two Rescuers—Adult Client

1. When second rescuer arrives, the first rescuer stops CPR after completing two ventilations and assesses for a carotid pulse for 5 seconds.

2. The second rescuer moves into the chest compression position.

3. If pulselessness continues, the first rescuer states "no pulse" and delivers one ventilation.

4. The second rescuer begins chest compression while counting out loud, " one and two and three and four and five and." The compression rate is 100/min.

5. The first rescuer gives two slow ventilations after 15 chest compressions. The first rescuer also assesses carotid pulse during chest compressions to evaluate effectiveness.

6. If second rescuer wishes to change positions, he or she states, "Change, one and two and three and four and five and."

PROCEDURE 35-3
ADMINISTERING CARDIOPULMONARY RESUSCITATION
(Continued)

Excellent	Satisfactory	Needs Practice		Comments

7. The first rescuer delivers the ventilation then moves into the chest compression position.

8. The second rescuer moves to the ventilator position and assesses for a carotid pulse for 5 seconds. If pulseless, resume CPR. Do not interrupt CPR for more than 7 seconds.

One Rescuer CPR—Infant and Child

1. Assess unresponsiveness.

2. If unresponsive, activate emergency response system (911) for children older than 8 years.

3. Place child on hard surface. Provide basic life support for 1 full minute before activating emergency medical system.

4. Open the airway using the head tilt/chin lift. Avoid overextension of head in infants.

5. Place you ear over child's mouth, and observe chest for rise. Listen, look, and feel for breathing. Perform Heimlich maneuver if airway obstruction from food or foreign object is suspected.

6. If breathlessness is determined, seal mouth and nose and ventilate twice (1-1.5 seconds for each breath). Observe for chest rise. In infants and small children, rescuer may need to place mouth over the mouth and nose to establish an airtight seal.

7. Assess pulselessness by palpating for carotid artery on near side in children older than 1 year. In infants younger than 1 year, assess brachial or femoral pulse for 5 seconds.

8. Begin chest compression if pulseless.

   a. For infant up to 1 year:

      (1) Visualize an imaginary line between the infant's nipples.

      (2) Place your index finger on the sternum just below this imaginary line.

      (3) Place your middle and fourth finger on sternum next to index finger.

   b. For child 1 to 8 years of age:

PROCEDURE 35-3
ADMINISTERING CARDIOPULMONARY RESUSCITATION
(Continued)

Excellent	Satisfactory	Needs Practice		Comments
—	—	—	(1) Placement of hand on sternum is the same as for adult CPR. Use heel of one hand to compress sternum 1 to 1½ inches 100 times/min.	
—	—	—	(2) Continue chest compressions, and ventilate at the rate of one breath to five compressions.	
—	—	—	(3) Continue CPR as for an adult.	

Name _____ Date _11/2/05_

Unit _____ Position _____

Instructor/Evaluator: _____ Position _____

PROCEDURE 37-1
MEASURING BLOOD GLUCOSE BY SKIN PUNCTURE

Goal: To monitor blood glucose levels for clients who are at risk for hypoglycemia or hyperglycemia.

Excellent	Satisfactory	Needs Practice		Comments
—	—	—	1. Have client wash hands with soap and warm water.	
—	—	—	2. Position client comfortably.	
—	—	—	3. Remove reagent strip from the container and handle according to the manufacturer's instructions.	
—	—	—	4. Place reagent strip with test pad up on a dry surface.	
—	—	—	5. Choose the finger to be punctured, massage gently, and hold in a dependent position.	
—	—	—	6. Wipe the puncture site with alcohol (or a povidone-iodine swab). Allow site to dry completely.	
—	—	—	7. Don gloves.	
—	—	—	8. Remove the cover of the lancet or autolet. Place the autolet against the side of the finger and push the release button. If using a lancet, hold it perpendicular to the site, and pierce the site quickly.	
—	—	—	9. Wipe the initial drop of blood with a cotton ball.	
—	—	—	10. Squeeze the puncture gently or massage the skin toward the site to obtain a large drop of blood. Hold reagent strip next to drop of blood, and allow blood to cover the test pad completely. Do not smear the blood. In some meters, bring the finger to the test site on the meter, and allow blood to drop onto appropriate area.	
—	—	—	11. Start timing (usually less than 60 seconds) using the glucose meter or a watch if the meter is not available.	
—	—	—	12. Following manufacturer's instruction, wipe the blood from the test pad with a cotton ball after the specified period of time.	
—	—	—	13. Place the reagent strip into the glucose meter. After the recommended period of time, read the results. For meters on which blood is placed directly, read the results at the designated time. If a glucose meter is not available, compare the color of the test pad with the color strip on the side of the reagent strip container.	

PROCEDURE 37-1
MEASURING BLOOD GLUCOSE BY SKIN PUNCTURE
(Continued)

Excellent

Satisfactory

Needs Practice

Comments

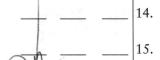

14. Turn off the glucose meter. Dispose of used equipment in the appropriate manner (needles in used needle receptacle).

15. Share test results with client, and record obtained values in the client's chart.

Name _Fallan Piyur_   Date _8/31/05_

Unit _____   Position _____

Instructor/Evaluator: _____   Position _____

Excellent	Satisfactory	Needs Practice	PROCEDURE 37-2 **ASSISTING AN ADULT WITH FEEDING**	Comments
			Goal: To maintain nutritional status.	
___	___	___	1. Prepare client's environment for meal:	
___		___	a. Remove urinals, bedpans, dressings, and trash.	
___		___	b. Ventilate or aerate room for unpleasant odors.	
___		___	c. Clean overbed table.	
___		___	2. Prepare client for meal:	
___		___	a. Help client to urinate or defecate.	
___		___	b. Help client to wash face and hands.	
___		___	c. Assist with oral hygiene.	
___			d. Help client to apply dentures, glasses, or special appliances.	
___			e. Assist to upright position in bed or chair.	
___		___	3. Wash your hands before touching meal tray.	
___		___	4. Check client's tray against diet order and with client's identification.	
___		___	5. Place tray on overbed table and move in front of client.	
___		___	6. Prepare tray. Open cartons, remove lids, season food, and cut food into bite-size pieces.	
___		___	7. Place napkin or towel under client's chin, and cover clothing.	
___			8. If client can feed self, leave and return in 10 to 15 minutes to determine if client is tolerating diet. (Do not leave client with overly hot liquids or food unless fully independent with feeding.)	
___	___	___	9. a. If client can sit in a chair but needs help to eat, sit in chair facing client.	
___		___	b. If client must remain in bed, you may stand to feed client.	
___		___	10. Allow client to choose the order in which he or she would like to eat. If client is visually impaired, identify the food on the tray.	
___	___	___	11. Warn client if food is hot or cold.	

PROCEDURE 37-2
ASSISTING AN ADULT WITH FEEDING
(Continued)

Excellent	Satisfactory	Needs Practice		Comments

12. Allow enough time between bites for adequate chewing and swallowing.

13. Offer liquids as requested or between bites. Use straw or special drinking cup if available.

14. Provide conversation during meal. Choose topic of interest to client. Reorient to current events or use meal as opportunity to educate on nutrition or discharge plans. Do **not** talk to clients who are relearning swallowing techniques; they need to concentrate.

15. Help client to wash hands and face, and perform oral hygiene after meal.

16. Assist to comfortable position and allow rest period. If at risk for aspiration, leave head of bed elevated for 30 minutes after eating.

17. Record fluids and amount of meal consumed, if ordered.

18. Remove and dispose of tray.

19. Wash hands.

passed
N Anderson RN MSN
8/31/03

Name _Fallon Pryor_   Date _10/26/05_

Unit _____   Position _____

Instructor/Evaluator: _JRiley RN_   Position _____

PROCEDURE 37-3
ADMINISTERING NUTRITION VIA NASOGASTRIC OR GASTROSTOMY TUBE

Goal: To provide enteral nutrition for comatose or semiconscious clients or to clients who cannot swallow or who have an esophageal obstruction.

Excellent	Satisfactory	Needs Practice		Comments

1. Wash hands.
2. Close room door or curtains around bed.
3. Explain procedure and purpose to client.
4. Help client to high Fowler's position by elevating head of bed at least 60 degrees or assisting to chair. If high Fowler's position is contraindicated, help client to a right side-lying position with head slightly elevated.
5. Confirm placement of tube in stomach:
   a. Withdraw sample of stomach contents, and check for low pH level.
   b. Attach 60 mL irrigation syringe to tube, and inject 10 mL of air while auscultating over epigastrium. Recognize that this may not be reliable index of tube placement when client has small-bore feeding tube.
   c. Aspirate all stomach contents, and measure for residual.
   d. If 100 mL or more than half of last feeding is aspirated, contact physician before proceeding with tube feeding. The feeding is usually held.
   e. Reinstill the aspirated gastric contents through tube into stomach.
6. Prepare correct amount and strength of formula at room temperature. (Optional: Add several drops of food coloring.)

Bolus of Intermittent Feeding

1. Remove plunger from irrigation syringe. Clamp gastric tubing and attach syringe. If using gavage bag, attach tubing to gastric tube.
2. Fill syringe or gavage bag with formula.

ADMINISTERING NUTRITION VIA NASOGASTRIC OR GASTROSTOMY TUBE (Continued)

Excellent	Satisfactory	Needs Practice		Comments

3. Allow feeding to flow in slowly over 10 to 15 minutes. If using syringe, raise and lower to adjust flow rate by gravity. Refill syringe as needed without disconnecting, avoiding air spaces in tubing. If gavage bag is used, hang bag on IV pole, and adjust flow rate with clamp on tubing.

4. Clamp tubing just as feeding is completing. Rinse tube with 30 to 60 mL tap water. Do not allow air to enter tubing.

5. Clamp gastric tube, and disconnect from syringe or gavage bag.

6. Have client remain in high Fowler's or elevated side-lying position for 30 to 60 minutes.

Continuous Feeding

1. Connect gavage tubing to gastric tube.

2. Hang gavage bag on IV pole.

3. Pour in desired amount of formula according to agency policy (usually amount to infuse in 3 hours).

4. a. Connect tubing to infusion pump.

   b. Set rate.

5. Check residual every 4 to 6 hours, according to agency policy. Then flush tubing with 30 to 60 mL water.

6. Have client remain in high Fowler's or slightly elevated side-lying position.

7. Wash any reusable equipment with soap and water. Change equipment every 24 hours or according to agency policy.

8. Wash hands.

9. Document procedure and observations.

Name Fallan Ryer

Date _____

Unit _____

Position _____

Instructor/Evaluator: O Turney RN ____

Position _____

Excellent	Satisfactory	Needs Practice	PROCEDURE 38-1 **CHANGING A DRY STERILE DRESSING** **Goal:** To protect wound from trauma and external contamination and to provide an opportunity to assess wound.	Comments
__	4/05	__	1. Close client's door or close curtains around bed. Explain procedure to client.	
__	__	__	2. Position client comfortably. Expose only wound area.	
__	__	__	3. Wash hands.	
__	__	__	4. Make a cuff on top of plastic bag, and place within easy reach of dressing table.	
__	__	__	5. Put on clean disposable gloves.	
__	__	__	6. Remove dressing from wound, and discard into plastic bag. If dressing adheres to wound, pour small amount of sterile saline on wound to loosen dressing.	
__	__	__	7. Remove and dispose of gloves. Wash hands.	
__	__	__	8. Set up sterile supplies:	
__	__	__	a. Open sterile towel, and hold it by edges.	
__	__	__	b. Place it on clean, flat surface without contaminating center of towel.	
__	__	__	c. Open dressing package(s) by peeling paper down to expose dressing. Let it fall onto sterile field.	
__	__	__	d. Open cleansing solution container, and pour solution into sterile cup.	
__	__	__	e. Open any supplies for wound irrigation, and set materials at side of sterile field. (Alternatively, open dressing packages and suture set carefully, allowing the inside of the packaging material to serve as the sterile field.)	
__	__	__	9. Don sterile gloves. Grasp applicators at nonabsorbent end, and dip into cleansing solution.	
__	__	__	10. Clean drainage from center of wound outward, using each applicator only once and discarding without placing applicator back into cleansing solution.	
__	__	__	11. Dry surrounding skin gently with gauze.	
__	__	__	12. Inspect incision for bleeding, inflammation, drainage, and healing. Note any areas of dehiscence.	

PROCEDURE 38-1
CHANGING A DRY STERILE DRESSING (Continued)

Excellent	Satisfactory	Needs Practice		Comments
			13. Apply sterile dressings one at a time over wound.	
			14. Wash hands.	
			15. Document procedure and observations.	

Name Fallan Pryor

Date _____

Unit _____

Position _____

Instructor/Evaluator: 6 Tierny Redon

Position _____

PROCEDURE 38-2
APPLYING SALINE-MOISTENED DRESSINGS

Excellent	Satisfactory	Needs Practice	**Goal:** To promote moist wound healing.	Comments
	11/05		1. Prepare client and remove dressing according to Steps 1 through 5 of Procedure 38-1. Forceps may be used to remove soiled dressing. If dressing adheres to underlying tissues, moisten with saline to loosen. Gently remove the dressing while assessing client's discomfort level.	
			2. Observe dressings for amount and characteristics of drainage. Note odor and color.	
			3. Observe wound for eschar, granulation tissue, or epithelial skin buds. Measure and record wound depth, diameter, and length.	
			4. Prepare sterile supplies. Open sterile instruments, sterile basin, solution, and dressings.	
			5. Place fine-mesh gauze into basin, and pour the ordered solution over mesh to saturate. For large wounds, warm ordered solution to body temperature.	
			6. Don sterile gloves.	
			7. Cleanse or irrigate wound as prescribed or with normal saline, moving from least to most contaminated areas.	
			8. Squeeze excess fluid from gauze dressing. Unfold and fluff out the dressing.	
			a. Gently pack moistened gauze into the wound.	
			b. If wound is deep, use forceps or cotton-tipped applicators to press gauze into all wound surfaces.	
			9. Apply several dry, sterile 4x4s over the wet gauze.	
			10. Place ABD pad over dry 4x4s.	
			11. Remove and dispose of sterile gloves.	
			12. Secure dressings with tape, Kerlix gauze, or Montgomery ties.	
			13. Assist client to a comfortable position.	
			14. Wash hands.	
			15. Document the procedure and observations.	

Name Fallan Pryur

Date _____

Unit _____

Position _____

Instructor/Evaluator: 6 Tierney RN on

Position _____

PROCEDURE 38-3
IRRIGATING A WOUND

Excellent	Satisfactory	Needs Practice	**Goal:** To cleanse wound by removing debris and exudate and promote wound healing.	Comments
___	___	___	1. Close door or curtains around bed. Explain procedure to client.	
___	___	___	2. Position client comfortably to allow irrigating solution to flow by gravity across wound and into a collection basin.	
___	___	___	3. Expose the wound area only. Place waterproof pad under client.	
___	___	___	4. Wash hands.	
___	___	___	5. Don mask, goggles, and gown if needed.	
___	___	___	6. Remove dressing and inspect wound. See Steps 1 through 4 of Procedure 38-2.	
___	___	___	7. Pour warmed irrigating solution into sterile basin.	
___	___	___	8. Open irrigating syringe, and place into basin with solution.	
___	___	___	9. Place second basin at distal end of wound to catch contaminated irrigating solution.	
___	___	___	10. Don sterile gloves.	
___	___	___	11. Fill irrigating syringe with solution. Holding syringe tip about 1 inch above the wound, gently flush all areas of wound. Continue flushing until solution draining into basin is clear.	
___	___	___	12. If wound is deep, attach latex or silicone catheter to syringe filled with irrigating solution. Gently insert catheter into wound and flush until returning solution is clear.	
___	___	___	13. Dry surrounding skin thoroughly.	
___	___	___	14. Apply sterile dressing.	
___	___	___	15. Remove and discard gloves.	
___	___	___	16. Secure dressing with tape or Montgomery straps.	
___	___	___	17. Assist client to comfortable position.	
___	___	___	18. Dispose of equipment. Retain remaining bottle of sterile solution for future irrigations. Mark date and time of opening on bottle for reference. Dispose according to agency policy.	

PROCEDURE 38-3
IRRIGATING A WOUND (Continued)

Excellent	Satisfactory	Needs Practice		Comments
			19. Wash hands.	
			20. Document procedure and observations.	

Name _____   Date _____

Unit _____   Position _____

Instructor/Evaluator: _____   Position _____

Excellent	Satisfactory	Needs Practice	PROCEDURE 38-4 **MAINTAINING A PORTABLE (HEMOVAC) WOUND SUCTION**	
			Goal: To facilitate healing by removing drainage from the incisional area.	**Comments**
___	___	___	1. Explain procedure, assist client to comfortable position, and pull curtains or close door.	
___	___	___	2. Wash hands. Don clean, disposable gloves.	
___	___	___	3. Expose Hemovac tubing and container while keeping client draped.	
___	___	___	4. Examine tubing and container for patency and suction seal.	
___	___	___	5. Open drainage plug.	
___	___	___	6. Pour drainage into a calibrated receptacle without contaminating drainage spout.	
___	___	___	7. Reestablish suction by placing reservoir on firm, flat surface. With drainage plug open, compress the unit and reinsert drainage plug.	
___	___	___	8. Remove and discard gloves.	
___	___	___	9. Return client to comfortable position.	
___	___	___	10. Measure drainage, and record amount, color, and other pertinent information.	

Name _____ Date _____

Unit _____ Position _____

Instructor/Evaluator: _____ Position _____

PROCEDURE 39-1
OBTAINING A WOUND CULTURE

Excellent	Satisfactory	Needs Practice		Comments

Goal: To identify organisms colonized within a wound so antibiotics sensitive to the microorganisms can be prescribed as needed.

—— —— ——   1. Identify client, and verify order for culture, noting site and type of culture.

—— —— ——   2. Wash hands, and apply clean disposable gloves.

—— —— ——   3. Remove soiled dressing. Observe drainage for amount, odor, and color.

—— —— ——   4. Clear and remove exudate from around wound with antiseptic swab.

Obtaining Aerobic Culture

—— —— ——   1. Perform Steps 1 to 4 above.

—— —— ——   2. Using sterile swab from culture tube, insert swab deep into area of active drainage. Rotate swab to absorb as much drainage as possible.

—— —— ——   3. Insert swab into culture tube, taking care not to touch the top or outside of tube.

—— —— ——   4. Crush ampule of medium, and close container securely.

—— —— ——   5. Continue with Step 4 below.

Obtaining Anaerobic Culture

—— —— ——   1. Perform Steps 1 to 4 at beginning of procedure.

—— —— ——   2. Using sterile swab from special anaerobic culture tube, insert swab deeply into draining body cavity.

—— —— ——   3. a. Rotate swab gently and remove. Quickly place swab into inner tube of collection container.

   b. *Alternative method*: Insert tip of syringe with needle removed into wound and aspirate 1 to 5 mL of exudate. Attach 21-gauge needle to syringe, expel all air, and inject exudate into inner tube of the culture container. Note: Drainage is sample from only one drainage site per culture swab. Repeat above steps for other drainage sites.

Excellent	Satisfactory	Needs Practice		Comments

PROCEDURE 39-1
OBTAINING A WOUND CULTURE (Continued)

___ ___ ___ 4. Label each culture tube, and send specimens with appropriate requisitions to the laboratory according to agency policy.

___ ___ ___ 5. Clean and apply sterile dressings to the wound as ordered.

___ ___ ___ 6. Remove and discard gloves. Wash hands.

___ ___ ___ 7. Assist client to comfortable position.

___ ___ ___ 8. Document all relevant information on client's chart. Include the location from which the specimen was taken and the date and time. Record the wound's consistency of drainage. Record how the client tolerated the procedure and any discomfort from the experience.

Name	Date
Unit	Position
Instructor/Evaluator:	Position

PROCEDURE 40-1
COLLECTING URINE SPECIMENS

Goal: To obtain a noncontaminated urine specimen for routine analysis or culture and sensitivity.

Columns: Excellent | Satisfactory | Needs Practice — Comments

Collecting Sterile Specimen From an Indwelling Catheter
1. Confirm physician's order, and verify the client.
2. Explain procedure to client.
3. Wash hands. Put on clean disposable gloves.
4. Position client so that catheter is accessible.
5. Drain urine from tubing into collection bag. Allow fresh urine to collect in tubing by clamping or bending tubing (2 mL of urine is sufficient for a culture and sensitivity specimen; 30 mL for urinalysis).
6. Cleanse aspiration port of drainage tubing with alcohol or Betadine swab.
7. Insert needle into aspiration port. Draw urine sample into syringe by gentle aspiration. Remove needle.
8. Transfer urine from syringe into a sterile specimen container.
9. Label container. Write date and time on laboratory requisition. Place in plastic biohazard bag for delivery to laboratory.
10. Send specimen to laboratory within 15 minutes, or place in specimen refrigerator. If specimen is for microbiology testing, do not refrigerate; send immediately.
11. Dispose of all contaminated supplies. Wash hands.
12. Document procedure and observations.

Self-Collecting Midstream Urine Specimen for a Woman
1. Instruct client how to cleanse urinary meatus and obtain urine specimen.
2. (Client) Wash hands.
3. Separate labia minora and cleanse perineum with cleansing agent, starting in front of the urethral meatus and moving swab toward the rectum.
4. Begin to urinate while continuing to hold labia apart. Allow first urine to flow into toilet.

PROCEDURE 40-1
COLLECTING URINE SPECIMENS (Continued)

Excellent Satisfactory Needs Practice

Comments

5. Hold specimen container under the urine stream and collect sample.

6. Remove specimen container, release hand from labia, seal container tightly, and finish voiding. Wash hands.

7. (Nurse) Put on disposable gloves to receive specimen container from the client. Dry outside of container with a paper towel.

8. Write date and time on laboratory specimen. Label the container, and place specimen container in biohazard bag.

9. Send specimen to laboratory within 15 minutes, or place in specimen refrigerator. If specimen is for microbiology testing, do not refrigerate; send immediately.

10. Dispose of all contaminated supplies. Wash hands.

Self-Collecting Midstream Urine Specimen for a Man

1. Confirm physician's order, and identify client.

2. Instruct client how to cleanse urinary meatus and obtain urine specimen.

3. (Client) Wash hands.

4. Cleanse end of penis with cleansing agent. If man is not circumcised, instruct him to retract foreskin to expose urinary meatus before cleansing and throughout specimen collection.

5. Begin to urinate, allowing urine to flow into toilet.

6. Pass specimen container into urine stream and collect sample.

7. Remove container, seal tightly, and finish voiding.

8. Follow Steps 7 to 10 above.

Collecting a Specimen From a Child Without Urinary Control

1. If parents are present, explain procedure to them.

2. Position child gently on back. Put on disposable gloves. Remove diaper.

3. Clean perineal-genital area gently with soap and water, followed by antiseptic.

4. For a girl: Separate labia and cleanse from front of urethral meatus toward rectum. Rinse with water and dry with cotton balls.

COLLECTING URINE SPECIMENS (Continued)

Excellent	Satisfactory	Needs Practice		Comments

5. For a boy: Cleanse penis and scrotum. If uncircumcised, retract foreskin and cleanse. Rinse with water and dry with gauze or cotton balls.

6. Remove paper backing from adhesive of collection bag.

7. Spread child's legs apart widely.

8. Apply collection bag over child's perineum, covering penis and scrotum on boy and urinary meatus and vagina of girl. Press adhesive to secure, starting at perineum and working outward.

9. Place a diaper on child loosely.

10. Remove gloves and wash hands.

11. Check the collector for urine every 15 minutes.

12. When urine specimen is obtained, glove again, and gently remove collection bag from skin, and empty urine into specimen container.

13. Tighten lid and cleanse outside of container if contaminated with urine, and place in plastic biohazard bag for transfer to laboratory.

14. Label the container. Write date and time on laboratory requisition.

15. Send specimen to laboratory within 15 minutes, or place in specimen refrigerator. Send immediately if specimen is for microbiology testing; do not refrigerate.

16. Dispose of all contaminated supplies. Wash hands.

17. Document that specimen was collected and sent.

114

Name _Fullor_____ Date _____

Unit _____ Position _____

Instructor/Evaluator: _____ Position _____

Excellent	Satisfactory	Needs Practice	PROCEDURE 40-2 **APPLYING A CONDOM CATHETER**	Comments
			Goal: To provide a means of collecting urine and controlling incontinence without the risk of infection that an indwelling urinary catheter imposes.	
—	—	—	1. Close room door or bedside curtain. Explain procedure to client.	
—	—	—	2. Wash hands.	
—	—	—	3. Assist client to supine position with only genitalia exposed.	
—	—	—	4. Put on disposable gloves. Wash client's genitals with soap and water. Towel dry.	
—	—	—	5. Trim or shave excess pubic hair from base of penis, if necessary.	
—	—	—	6. Apply thin film of skin protector on penis shaft. Allow to dry for 30 seconds.	
—	—	—	7. Peel paper backing from both sides of adhesive liner and wrap spirally around penis shaft.	
—	—	—	8. Place funnel end of pre-rolled condom against glans of penis. Unroll sheath the length of the penis, over the adhesive liner. Some brands of condom catheters are held in place with a Velcro strap over the condom catheter.	
—	—	—	9. Attach funnel end of condom to collection system. Tape may be used to secure the connection below level of condom, avoiding kinks or loops in tubing.	
—	—	—	10. Discard used supplies. Remove and discard gloves. Wash hands.	
—	—	—	11. Observe penis 15 to 30 minutes after application of condom for swelling or changes in skin color. (If too tight, remove and reapply larger size.)	
—	—	—	12. Document procedure and observations.	

Name _Falan Pryor_   Date _9/28/05_

Unit _____   Position _____

Instructor/Evaluator: _____   Position _____

<table>
<tr><th>Excellent</th><th>Satisfactory</th><th>Needs Practice</th><th>PROCEDURE 40-3
INSERTING A STRAIGHT OR INDWELLING URINARY CATHETER</th><th></th></tr>
<tr><td></td><td></td><td></td><td>**Goal:** To monitor urinary function, relieve bladder distension, obtain sterile urine specimen, or provide a means for irrigating the bladder.</td><td>**Comments**</td></tr>
</table>

1. Verify physician's order, and identify the client.
2. Explain procedure and rationale to client.
3. Provide client with opportunity to perform personal perineal/penile hygiene. Assist client as necessary.
4. Wash your hands.

Inserting Catheter for a Woman

1. Position in dorsal recumbent position. Externally rotate thighs. Side-lying is alternate position.
2. Set up light source.
3. Open catheterization tray, maintaining asepsis.
4. Slide sterile drape under client's buttocks, grasping corners of drape. Ask client to lift hips so drape can be positioned.
5. Don sterile gloves.
6. Open sterile lubricant, and lubricate catheter tip. Open cleansing solution, and pour over half of the sterile cotton balls. Open sterile specimen container. Inflate balloon with prefilled syringe to check for defective balloon. Aspirate fluid back into syringe and leave attached.
7. Place nondominant hand on labia minora and gently spread to expose urinary meatus. Visualize exact location of meatus. During cleansing and catheter insertion, do not allow labia to close over meatus until after catheter is inserted.
8. Using sterile hand, pick up antiseptic solution-saturated cotton ball with sterile forceps.
9. Cleanse urinary meatus with one downward stroke. Discard cotton ball. Repeat this step three or four times.
10. Use forceps and dry cotton balls to absorb excess antiseptic solution.

Comments: _9/27/05_

PROCEDURE 40-3
INSERTING A STRAIGHT OR INDWELLING URINARY CATHETER (Continued)

Excellent	Satisfactory	Needs Practice		Comments

11. Place distal catheter end into sterile basin. With sterile hand, pick up catheter approximately 3 inch from tip and dip into sterile lubricant (2% lidocaine gel may be used). Place distal catheter end into sterile basin.

12. Gently insert catheter into urethra approximately 2 inch until urine begins to drain. If no urine appears, have client cough, or reposition catheter by rotating. Have client take slow, deep breaths during catheter insertion.

13. Insert catheter an additional 1 inch or 2.5 cm. If catheter enters vagina by mistake, leave it there as a landmark. Insert second catheter into meatus.

14. Obtain urine specimen in sterile container, if ordered.

15. If using straight catheter: Allow bladder to empty, then remove straight catheter. Measure urine.

16. If using indwelling catheter: Inflate the retention balloon with the prefilled syringe. Check to ensure placement by gently pulling on catheter.

17. Connect distal end of catheter to drainage bag (may prefer to connect prior to catheter insertion).

18. Tape catheter securely with 1-inch tape to inner thigh with enough give so it will not pull when moving the legs.

19. Attach drainage bag to bed frame, ensuring that tubing does not fall into dependent loops or that side rails do not interfere with drainage system.

20. Remove gloves. Wash hands.

21. Record time procedure was complete, size of catheter inserted, amount and color of urine, and any adverse client responses.

Inserting Catheter for a Man

1. Position client in supine position with only genitalia exposed.

2. Drape legs to mid-thigh with bath blanket or sheet.

3. Open catheterization tray.

4. Put on sterile gloves. Open sterile lubricant and lubricate catheter tip. Open cleansing solution and pour over half of the sterile cotton balls. Open sterile specimen container. Inflate balloon with prefilled syringe to check for defective balloon. Aspirate fluid back into syringe and leave attached.

PROCEDURE 40-3
INSERTING A STRAIGHT OR INDWELLING URINARY CATHETER (Continued)

Comments

5. Place the fenestrated drape over the client's genitalia.
6. With nondominant hand, hold penis at a 90-degree angle to his body. If client is not circumcised, pull back foreskin with this hand to visualize the urethral meatus.
7. Using the sterile hand, pick up antiseptic solution-soaked cotton ball with sterile forceps.
8. Cleanse the urinary meatus with one downward stroke, or use a circular motion from meatus to base of penis. Discard cotton ball. Repeat this step at least three to four times.
9. Use forceps to pick up one dry cotton ball to dry the meatus.
10. With sterile hand, pick up the catheter approximately 3 inches from the tip and lubricate catheter generously. Place distal catheter end into sterile basin.
11. Gently insert catheter into urethra (approximately 8 inch) until urine begins to drain.
12. Insert catheter an additional 1 inch or 2.5 cm.
13. If using an indwelling catheter, inflate the retention balloon with the prefilled syringe.
14. Check for placement by gently pulling on catheter.
15. Connect distal end of catheter to drainage bag if necessary.
16. Tape catheter securely with 1-inch tape to the abdomen.
17. In the uncircumcised male, gently replace the foreskin over the glans.
18. Attach drainage bag to bed frame, coiling tubing to ensure that tubing does not fall into dependent loops.
19. Wash hands.
20. Record time procedure was complete, size of catheter, amount and color of urine, and any adverse client responses.

Removing an Indwelling Catheter
1. Wash hands.
2. Don clean, disposable gloves.
3. Clamp catheter (optional).

PROCEDURE 40-3
INSERTING A STRAIGHT OR INDWELLING URINARY CATHETER (Continued)

Excellent	Satisfactory	Needs Practice		Comments
			4. Insert hub of syringe into balloon inflation tube of catheter, and draw out all liquid.	
			5. Ask client to breathe in and out deeply. Pinch gently and remove catheter as client exhales.	
			6. Assist client to cleanse and dry genitals.	
			7. Measure and document urine in drainage bag and time of catheter removal.	
			8. Wash hands.	

Name Fallon Pryor   Date 9/28/05

Unit _____   Position _____

Instructor/Evaluator: _____   Position _____

Excellent	Satisfactory	Needs Practice	

PROCEDURE 41-1
ASSESSING STOOL FOR OCCULT BLOOD

Goal: To screen clients who have or are at risk for gastrointestinal bleeding.

Comments

1. Identify client. Ask client to void before collecting stool specimen.
2. Assist client onto bedpan, onto commode, or into bathroom. Provide privacy, and leave call bell within reach.
3. When client has passed stool and is clean and comfortable, don disposable gloves, and obtain small amount of stool with tongue blade or wooden applicator.

9/28/05

Hemoccult Slide Test

1. Open flap of slide, and apply a very thin smear of stool taken from center of the specimen onto first window.
2. Using second applicator, obtain a second sample from a different area of stool. Smear thinly on second window of slide.
3. Close slide cover. Open flap on reverse side, and apply two drops of Hemoccult developing solution onto each window.
4. Wait 30 to 60 seconds. Read test results.

Test With Hematest Tablets

1. Apply small smear of stool onto guaiac filter paper.
2. Place Hematest tablet on stool sample.
3. Apply two to three drips of water onto Hematest tablet. Hold paper so water runs onto it.
4. Read test results within 2 minutes by observing color of guaiac paper
5. Remove gloves, wash hands, and document findings.

Name _Fallon Prye_   Date _10/19/05_

Unit _____   Position _____

Instructor/Evaluator: _N. Anderson RN_   Position _____

Excellent	Satisfactory	Needs Practice	PROCEDURE 41-2 **ADMINISTERING AN ENEMA**	Comments

Goal: To relieve gas, constipation, or fecal impaction or to cleanse bowel in preparation for diagnostic tests.

1. Assemble needed equipment in one place; then provide privacy by closing curtains or room door.
2. Identify client. Position of left side (Sims' position) with right knee flexed.
3. Put on disposable gloves. Place waterproof towel under client's buttocks.
4. Cover client with bath blanket, exposing only the rectum.

Large-Volume Enema

1. See Steps 1 to 4.
2. Fill enema bag with 750 to 1000 mL lukewarm solution (105° to 110°F; for child, use 500 mL or less at 100°F).
3. Open clamp on tubing, and allow solution to flow through tubing to remove the air. Reclamp tubing.
4. Lubricate 2 to 3 inches of tip of rectal tube with water-soluble lubricant.
5. Separate the buttocks to visualize the anus. Observe for external hemorrhoids. Ask client to take a slow, deep breath. Gently insert the rectal tube (3-4 inches in the adult), directing the tip toward the umbilicus.
6. Continue holding the tube in the rectum. With other hand, open the clamp and allow solution to slowly enter the client. Raise container 18 inches above the anus, allowing solution to flow slowly over 5 to 10 minutes. If client complains of cramping or pain, have client breathe deeply and lower bag until sensation stops.
7. Reclamp tubing when desired amount of solution has infused.
8. Remove tube gently and have client squeeze buttocks together firmly for several minutes.
9. Have client retain solution as long as possible.
10. Assist client to bathroom, commode, or bedpan. Place call bell within reach. Provide privacy until all solution has been expelled.

PROCEDURE 41-2
ADMINISTERING AN ENEMA (Continued)

Excellent	Satisfactory	Needs Practice		Comments
			11. Visually inspect character of the feces and solution. If client is to have enemas until clear, allow client to rest and then repeat as necessary.	
			12. Assist client into comfortable position. Assist with cleansing as needed. Provide materials for client to wash hands. Open windows or provide air freshener if needed. Clean and dispose of equipment as necessary. Remove gloves and wash hands.	

Small-Volume Enema

1. See Steps 1 to 4 at beginning of procedure.

2. Remove protective cap from prelubricated catheter tip. You may add more lubricant if necessary.

3. Separate the buttocks to visualize the anus. Observe for hemorrhoids, and gently insert rectal tip into rectum, directing tip toward the umbilicus.

4. Squeeze bottle to empty contents into the rectum and colon (approximately 240 mL).

5. Maintain pressure on the enema container until you withdraw it from the rectum.

6. Continue same as with large-volume enema (see Steps 9 to 12).

Name _____   Date _____

Unit _____   Position _____

Instructor/Evaluator: _____   Position _____

Excellent	Satisfactory	Needs Practice	
			PROCEDURE 41-3 **INSERTING A NASOGASTRIC TUBE**
			Goal: To decompress the stomach to relieve pressure and prevent vomiting, to deliver enteral feedings, to provide a means to irrigate the stomach, or to obtain gastric specimen. **Comments**
___	___	___	1. Identify client and explain procedure.
___	___	___	2. Provide privacy by closing curtains or room door. Raise bed to high Fowler's position, cover chest with towel, and place emesis basin nearby.
___	___	___	3. Wash hands, and put on gloves. Determine length of tubing to be inserted by measuring nasogastric tube from tip of ear lobe to tip of nose, then to tip of xiphoid process. Mark tubing with adhesive tape or note striped markings already on tube.
___	___	___	4. Lubricate tip of tube with water-soluble lubricant.
___	___	___	5. Gently insert tube into nostril. Advance toward posterior pharynx.
___	___	___	6. Have client tilt head forward and encourage client to drink water slowly. Advance tube without using force as client swallows. Advance tube until desired insertion length is reached.
___	___	___	7. Temporarily tape the tube to client's nose; then assess placement of tube:
___	___	___	a. Aspirate gastric content with 20- to 50-mL syringe.
___	___	___	b. Auscultate over epigastrium while injecting 10 to 20 mL air into nasogastric tube.
___	___	___	c. If feeding tube is placed, confirmation of placement is required before any feeding is administered.
___	___	___	8. If placement in stomach is not verified, untape tube, advance tube 5 cm, and repeat assessment in Step 7.
___	___	___	9. Secure tube by taping to bridge of client's nose. Anchor tubing to client's gown.
___	___	___	10. Clamp end of tubing or attach to suction, as ordered by health care provider.
___	___	___	11. Wash hands, provide for client's comfort, and remove equipment.

INSERTING A NASOGASTRIC TUBE (Continued)

Excellent	Satisfactory	Needs Practice		Comments
——	——	——	12. Establish and document a nursing plan for daily care of nasogastric tube:	
——	——	——	a. Inspect nostril for irritation.	
——	——	——	b. Cleanse nostril frequently.	
——	——	——	c. Change adhesive as required to prevent skin irritation or pressure sores on nostril from tube.	
——	——	——	d. Increase frequency of oral care because clients with nasogastric tubes often mouth breathe and may be NPO.	
——	——	——	13. Document procedure and observations.	

Name Fallan Pryor   Date 9/28/05

Unit _____   Position _____

Instructor/Evaluator: _____   Position _____

PROCEDURE 41-4
APPLYING A FECAL OSTOMY POUCH

Excellent	Satisfactory	Needs Practice		Comments

Goal: To provide a means to contain drainage and odors from a fecal ostomy.

1. Identify client and provide privacy. Don disposable gloves. Client may perform procedure on self without gloves.
2. Gently remove old appliance. If disposable, discard. If reusable, set aside for washing.
3. Wash skin thoroughly around stoma with skin cleanser or soap and water.
4. Rinse skin thoroughly and blot dry.
5. Observe condition of peristomal skin, the stoma, and the sutures. Teach client to make these observations daily.
6. Prepare clean pouch. Measure stoma and trace circle $1/8$ inch larger than stoma on adhesive paper backing. Cut stoma pattern.
7. Prepare skin barrier. Measure stoma and cut hole in barrier the same size as stoma. Be sure edges are rounded.
8. If stoma is located in abdominal crease or skin is irregular, use paste barrier to fill the irregularity.
9. Apply protective skin barrier.
   a. Peel paper backing off wafer and center stoma in hole.
   b. Place on abdomen, pressing lightly over all areas of the barrier to promote adhesion with skin surfaces.
10. Attach drainable pouch to skin barrier. (Some equipment attaches by plastic flange that snaps in place; other models adhere through self-adherent tape that is exposed after protective paper backing is removed.) Tug gently or inspect for secure fit.
11. Frame every edge of the faceplate with hypoallergenic tape.
12. Fold over bottom edge of pouch and clamp.
13. Dispose of old appliance. Clean and store any reusable supplies. Wash hands. Document noted observations.

Name _____ Date _____

Unit _____ Position _____

Instructor/Evaluator: _____ Position _____

Excellent	Satisfactory	Needs Practice	

PROCEDURE 44-1
REMOVING CONTACT LENSES

Goal: To remove contact lenses in the event the client is unable to do so.

Comments

Removing Hard Contact Lenses

___ ___ ___ 1. Wash hands with soap and warm water.

___ ___ ___ 2. Position client comfortably in sitting position if possible.

___ ___ ___ 3. Pull the client's upper and lower lid apart and pull tautly toward the lateral side.

___ ___ ___ 4. Ask client to blink, and the lens should pop out into your hand.

___ ___ ___ 5. Alternatively: Use lens suction cup, especially for clients who cannot consciously assist with removal.

Removing Soft Contact Lenses

___ ___ ___ 1. Wash hands with soap and warm water.

___ ___ ___ 2. Position client comfortably in a sitting position if possible.

___ ___ ___ 3. Ask client to look upward and inward. Pull down on the lower lid and place your index finger on the lower edge of the lens, moving it onto the white part of the eye.

___ ___ ___ 4. Gently grasp lens between thumb and index finger to release the suction of the lens. The lens will fold over and be easily removed. Gently roll the lens, using normal saline as needed, to separate the lens and return it to its normal form.

Name _____   Date _____

Unit _____   Position _____

Instructor/Evaluator: _____   Position _____

Excellent	Satisfactory	Needs Practice		Comments
			PROCEDURE 44-2 **ASSISTING ADULT WITH INSERTING A HEARING AID**	
			Goal: To maintain hearing status by assisting with insertion of hearing aid.	
___	___	___	1. Check to be sure that the battery is functional. Hold hearing aid in hand and turn up the volume until you hear a "feedback" whistle.	
___	___	___	2. Inspect hearing aid to be sure that the tubing and ear mold are intact and not cracked or broken. The opening of the ear mold should be free of cerumen.	
___	___	___	3. With volume turned down, insert the ear mold into the ear canal, twisting slightly for a snug fit.	
___	___	___	4. Secure the battery behind the ear, if of that type.	
___	___	___	5. Turn the volume up slowly while speaking to the client in a normal voice tone. Ask client to let you know when the sound level is comfortable.	